MODERN MEDICINE IN THE HOLY LAND

MODERN MEDICINE IN THE HOLY LAND

Pioneering British Medical Services in Late Ottoman Palestine

YARON PERRY
EFRAIM LEV

Tauris Academic Studies
LONDON • NEW YORK

Published in 2007 by Tauris Academic Studies, an imprint of I.B.Tauris & Co Ltd
6 Salem Road, London W2 4BU
175 Fifth Avenue, New York NY 10010
www.ibtauris.com

In the United States of America and Canada distributed by Palgrave Macmillan a division of St. Martin's Press, 175 Fifth Avenue, New York NY 10010

International Library of Colonial History 8

ISBN: 978 1 84511 489 3

A full CIP record for this book is available from the British Library
A full CIP record is available from the Library of Congress

Library of Congress Catalog Card Number: available

Printed and bound by Thomson Press India Limited
From camera-ready copy edited and supplied by the authors

CONTENTS

LIST OF ILLUSTRATIONS

Sources: fig. 1 - *Jewish Intelligence*, July 1845, opposite p. 241; fig. 2 - *Jewish Missionary Intelligence*, July 1897, p. 109; fig. 3- Ibid., p. 101; figs. 4, 7 – Yaron Perry; figs. 5, 6, 8, 9, 10, 18 - slides collection, Schick's Library, Christ Church, Jerusalem; fig. 11 - slides collection, St Albans Archive; fig. 12 - *JMI*, July 1899, p. 99; figs. 13, 14, 15 – Ibid., July 1897, p. 102; fig. 16 – Ibid., June 1914, p. 86; fig. 17 – Ibid., June 1907, p. 93; fig. 19 - Israeli Trust of the Anglican Church Archive, Jerusalem, Medical diaries, p. 386.

The authors wish to thank Mr Kelvin Crombie and Mr Avraham Perrodin of Christ Church, Jerusalem, for providing photographs no. 2,3,5,6,8,9,10, 12,14,15,17,18

PREFACE

The book placed before us sums up a five-year research project that began in the courtyard of the English Mission Hospital in the Galilean city of Safed. There, facing the impressive but abandoned building marked by the continual ravages of time, both of us, a historian and a biologist, tried to reconstruct one day in the life of the medical institution that had been set up more than a century ago. We tried to restore to life, if only for a moment, the feverish tumult associated with a medical institution of this size. We tried to gaze into the sombre faces of the doctors and nurses hard at work. We wanted to visualize the grateful expressions on the faces of the many patients that visited the hospital from day to day.

Years went by, during which we were engaged in studying the miserable sanitary conditions and the widespread ailments that were a common part of daily life among the inhabitants of the Holy Land. We laid bare the difficult process of establishing medical institutions hampered by the obstacles created by the Ottoman authorities. We learnt about the heroic efforts, sometimes at the cost of their lives, by doctors of different nationalities and various faiths. We examined the innovative methods of treatment that were used and the medicinal substances which had contributed so much to public health in the Holy Land. We investigated the conflicts of interest between the various European powers, between the

Christian churches within themselves and the Jewish communities throughout the country. We noted the fierce competition that developed as a result of these conflicting interests, whether national, inter-religious, inter-communal or interpersonal. Interests concentrated within such a narrow geographical region, so inferior in strategic, economic and military value and so far removed from the capitals of the powers involved. It was this competition that found expression in an intensive medical activity that entirely transformed the Holy Land.

So far, two pioneering studies have touched on a few aspects treated in this book. In 1983, Norbert Schwake surveyed the medical institutions in Jerusalem, and in 1998 Nissim Levy reviewed the initiation of medical practice and institutions in the Land of Israel. They were followed by several other researchers such as Samuel Kottek, Shmuel Nissan, Shifra Shvarts, Zalman Greenberg, Nakhle Bishara, Zvi Shilony, Rivka Izhaki and Avraham Morgenstern. These important articles dealt, in a limited manner, either with some specific aspect or a certain medical institution during the brief period in which it functioned.

This study documents a unique phenomenon of worldwide proportions. The book offers the reader a complete and comprehensive picture, from the year 1825 until the First World War, of a pioneering medical enterprise by the English Mission in Palestine. It examines the historical, economic, social and missionary aspects, and for the first time, the outstanding medical aspects of the 'revolution' that occurred in the Land of Israel. It discloses in detail the biographies of the main personages engaged in medical work, and their significant contributions to the historical, archaeological, botanical, zoological, geographical, hydrological, theological and linguistic research of the Holy Land. It surveys the development of the main hospitals founded in response to the construction of the English Mission hospitals. This development laid the foundations for modern medicine in the Land of Israel.

This book is dedicated to the physicians of various nations and faiths who were active in the Land of Israel during the nineteenth century. These pioneers improved medical conditions and relieved the sufferings of the country's inhabitants by building up a system of medical treatment and care that provided the basis for contemporary medicine, and they made considerable personal sacrifices in doing so. The book is also dedicated to the Israeli researchers – historians, doctors and biologists – who are now examining the history of medicine in various periods. This group of people, working cooperatively, are educating generations of students who follow them in this same spirit.

We would like to express our gratitude to our three readers for their editing job and helpful remarks: David Fruchtman, Israel, Dr David Wright, Scotland, Linda Barron, Israel, and the other anonymous readers.

Yaron Perry and Efraim Lev
Zichron Yaakov, Israel
2007

INTRODUCTION

Historical introduction

At the beginning of the nineteenth century the Land of Israel was still enveloped in medieval darkness, in contrast with the European world that had experienced the Renaissance centuries before. The brief period of conquest by Napoleon Bonaparte (1769-1821) in the spring of 1799 did not create any far-reaching changes. After the French had gone, the waning Ottoman Empire resumed control over the country, and continued as in the past to hinder foreign activities in the Holy Land. Yet the Napoleonic expedition was significant in making Christian Europe aware that the mighty Turkish conqueror had become a broken reed and that the continuation of Muslim rule over the Land of Israel was not assured. Hopes arose among Christian believers that it would be possible, after five centuries of absence, to take possession once again of the holy places in Jerusalem.

However, the actual turning point in European access to the area took place only during the 1830s. Muhammad Ali (1769-1848), the Governor of Egypt and a subject of the Sultan Mahmud II, launched his campaign of conquest into the heart of Ottoman Empire, overrunning the Land of Israel on his way. In order to appease the European Powers which, except for France, had not granted international recognition to his conquests, and regarded the threat to Constantinople as undermining the status quo, the Egyptians conducted a conciliatory policy towards the non-Muslim population in the Land of Israel. Within the framework of their liberal policies, the Egyptians granted equal rights to the Jews and

Christians in the country, opened the gates and allowed foreigners to settle there. In their desire to prove to the Christian world that their rule was preferable to their Turkish predecessors, the Egyptians laid the groundwork for wide-ranging European activities that completely altered the state of the country.

In 1839, the Turks began a military campaign to drive Muhammad Ali from the territories he had conquered at the beginning of that decade. The campaign was unsuccessful, the Ottoman army was beaten, and the Egyptians once again threatened Constantinople. In order to prevent the collapse of the Empire and the turmoil that would occur in Europe regarding what was called 'The Eastern Question', the European Powers met in London to discuss the ways in which they could extricate themselves from the crisis. At the end of the discussions, Britain, Russia, Austria and Prussia banded together to drive the Egyptians out of the Land of Israel. Disputes that arose between these Powers over competition for possession of the Land of Israel, prevented them from establishing Christian rule over the Holy Land. It was this competition, rather than the power of Constantinople, that re-installed Muslim rule of the country for nearly eighty more years. However, the Ottomans did not ignore the expectations raised in the Christian world that the new rulers would adopt the reforms introduced by their Egyptian predecessors and would maintain the equality of rights granted to the non-Muslims in the Land of Israel. [1]

Thus, after the return of the Turks, European clergymen and diplomats, settlers and researchers, travelers and adventurers visited the Holy Land in greater security and comfort, and in greater numbers.

Protestant England showed little interest in the Land of Israel at the beginning of the nineteenth century. Unlike France, Russia and Austria, England was almost totally indifferent toward the holy places in the country, and no British subjects or members of the Protestant faith were living there under its protection. British concerns focused on efforts to prevent the competing European Powers from staking claims to the country that might endanger Britain's vital interests in the region. Even the first intervention of Britain and the assistance it provided the Turks in blocking

Napoleon's advance in the East was not to acquire a foothold in the Land of Israel, but only to prevent France from endangering Britain's advance eastward. However, this strategic consideration was accompanied from the very first with indications of special support for the ties of the Jewish people to the Holy Land and for the idea of 'The Restoration of the Jews'.

The main tenets of faith, which had taken hold among many Protestants, stated that the Second Coming of Jesus Christ was imminent, and his advent would herald the utopian epoch of the Millennium. An important factor in this body of faith and a condition for the fulfilment of this apocalyptic vision was the return of the Jews to the land of their fathers and their immediate conversion, or alternatively, their recognition of the Messianic claims of the Christian Saviour.[2]

Those who were prompted by a deep sympathy for the Jewish people which they had derived from the Holy Scriptures, considered the idea of their restoration as a means of atonement for the sins committed by the Church against the Jews. There were also some self interested factions who considered the Jews a useful tool in the process of hastening the return of the Messiah. In any event, both these groups gave active support to the return of the Jews to their homeland, either by attempting to make the Land of Israel a habitable place, or by promoting the welfare of the Jews living in Palestine in order to attract their Jewish brethren in the Diaspora. Either way, their main purpose was still defined by the desire to bring the Jews closer to Jesus and thereby also to 'redemption'. On the basis of this belief, many societies were established around the world with the aim of spreading the missionary gospel among the Jews. The most prominent among all these was the 'London Jews Society for Promoting Christianity Amongst the Jews'.

History of the London Jews Society

In 1809, Christian Friedrich Frey (1771-1850), a converted Jew and native of Meinstockheim near Kitzingen in the duchy of Franconia, founded 'The London Jews Society for Promoting Christianity Amongst the Jews' that aimed to spread the Gospel among the Jews of East London.[3] Missionary activity in those days was conducted mainly in London, and at the end of the second decade of the nineteenth century the Society thought it was high time to explore additional fields of activity outside the British Isles, mainly in the Mediterranean littoral and in Palestine.

During the years 1820-1840, the London Jews Society dispatched a dozen missionaries to Palestine, but various obstacles prevented them from settling permanently in Jerusalem in the 1820s. The only Europeans who were allowed to remain in Palestine under Turkish rule were the keepers of the Christian Holy Places. European Protestants as a rule, were regarded with great suspicion by the Ottoman regime in Palestine, as well as by the Catholic Church, the Greek-Orthodox and the Armenians who had maintained a hold in the Holy Places in Jerusalem for centuries. Protestant attempts to settle in Jerusalem failed, as they had not been present in Palestine prior to the Ottoman conquest in 1516, and therefore were not recognized by the Ottoman rulers.

However, the conquest of Palestine by the Egyptians at the beginning of the 1830s, and their pursuit of a different policy, allowed the missionaries to establish a foothold in Jerusalem. The new era began with the initiative of John Nicolayson (1803-1856), the Society's emissary, native of Lügumkloster in Schleswig.[4] He settled down on October 22, 1833 with his family in Jerusalem and established a permanent Mission Station. Nicolayson wrote in his memoirs:

> Only when the Egyptian army under the command of Ibrahim Pasha had entered Palestine was I able to return with my family from Malta to Beirut, and after the conquest of Acre and complete [Egyptian] control over the country ... I managed] to settle for the first time in Jerusalem ... Therefore it should be noted that the first permanent settlement of the [Protestant] Mission in Jerusalem itself began only in 1833.[5]

It was only then, and especially after the re-establishment of the Turkish regime, with the help of England in 1840, that British missionaries began to thrive in Palestine.

The Mission

Leaders of the nineteenth century missionary societies, mainly the English Protestant, shared the concept that by means of the physician's art, an opening could be provided for the teaching of the Gospel in highly favourable circumstances. The main ideas and aims of mission were based upon three main pillars: a. attracting notice, b. disarming prejudice, and c. enlisting sympathy. Some argued that medical work was the most efficient way to achieve these aims and fulfill these purposes. The medical missions were, according to some: 'advertisement without quackery', a simple and easy road to confidence, frequently the conferring of benefits which were unmistakable and highly valued. People could be touched where they were most susceptible, either as to personal health or family affection.[6]

Medical missions were established:

> only where no European doctors are resident, or likely to be; where disease is widely prevalent, and yet is treated empirically by native doctors without education or skill; where men die in hundreds, of curable diseases, and where a trained physician and surgeon would be a great practical boon to a poor community...

To sum up the significant role of medical mission, Dr James Elder Cumming (1830-1909), a Scottish clergyman and scholar, wrote that it must be remembered that the spiritual work is the end in view and the practice of medicine the means to reach it. 'It is a mission to souls, carried on by means or with the assistance, medical skill'.[7]

Only pure faith could have enabled the missionaries to withstand the vicissitudes caused by the harassing journey, the harsh living conditions of the places where they worked, and the isolation and distance from the sources of their faith in London. To this should be added the hostility of the Jewish communities – and in some places, certainly in the Land of Israel, even physical malevolence by the local Ottoman authorities. The patrons of the London Jews Society foresaw these difficulties, and as a result, they occasionally published pamphlets of several pages entitled General Instructions.[8] In the opening pages of the booklet published in 1850, a few sketches were drawn of what might be encountered by the emissaries in their target countries, such as, for example, the necessity to foresee

> acts of villainy that the European eye is not usually aware of; the need to take part in futile and meaningless debates with the local population; the stamina to cope with periods of inactivity, idleness, feelings of impatience, disappointment and failure.[9]

The leaders of the London Jews Society faced problems in recruiting missionaries who were capable of enduring such conditions. When the candidates for the position of missionaries were finally able to meet a long list of demands, they had to spend a few years in training institutions. It was only when they passed the final exams successfully that they were given authority to serve as regular missionaries.

It seems that one can characterize a typical missionary by his form of activity, at least during the first decades of the London Jews Society's existence. In most cases, the missionaries who were sent to the Land of Israel were multi-lingual, with emphasis on the German language in order to make it easier for them to converse with the Yiddish-speaking *Ashkenazi* community. The Society considered it an added advantage to have missionaries who were Jewish converts, making good use of them to arouse the faith of the target population. The rabbis of Jerusalem were not unaware of the relative success of these converts, and they proclaimed that:

> It is no secret matter that the most dangerous among the inciters are the 'apostates' who are the seed of Jacob. Verily, the best among the propagandists, instigators, and seducers in the Land of Israel and in the East, have been, and still are, the apostates who have become the disciples of missionary institutions in Jerusalem and Safed.[10]

Before the missionary arrived at his post, exact information was collected for him, as far as this was possible, regarding the composition of the Jewish community and the conditions of the local regime. This was done by excursions conducted in advance and reliance on the reports of travellers who had visited the place. After setting out on his mission, the missionary stayed in a nearby mission station in order to acquire more recent information, and in some cases, also to learn the language of that place and to become acquainted with the living conditions and the climate. As soon as he had reached his destination, the missionary would begin by walking through the city squares to arouse the interest of the inhabitants while trying to distribute pamphlets and to sell copies of the Jewish Bible and the New Testament. At the same time he would often pay good money to hire the services of one of the rabbis to be his teacher in Hebrew and guide him in studying the scriptures, so that one day he could use the relationship between them to gain access to the community itself. Finally the missionary would conduct lengthy, in-depth discussions with the rabbis and the local people on the verities of the Old Testament as against the New Testament, in the hope of persuading and perhaps even converting them eventually.

Various means were employed by the missionaries in their attempts to bring the Jews of Palestine closer to the Christian faith. First and foremost, they tried to expose them to the Christian scriptures. They set up a book depôt, where texts sacred to Judaism and Christianity were available for sale or distribution. Converted Jews were employed in this repository to read the New Testament to passers by in their own language. Another way to reach the hearts of the Jews was to set up a secular school system with the intention of influencing the children of the community first, and through them reaching their parents. The members of the Society took advantage of the fact that Jewish youngsters received only religious education in their communities, and offered them the acceptable alternative of a free educational system.

But the institutions which proved to be the most successful in religious conversion were the hospitals of the London Jews Society whose leaders were well aware of the poor standard of health among the Palestinian Jews and of the total lack of Jewish medical facilities. In the early stages of their missionary activities they already dispatched physicians to their mission stations, opened dispensaries for the sale and distribution of medicines and clinics to provide first-aid services. Once the Mission Stations were well established in Palestine and the real medical needs of the local population were realised, hospitals were built in Jerusalem and Safed. The gratitude felt by the Jewish patients towards the missionaries who served in the medical institutions made them far more receptive and willing to become familiar with the Christian scriptures. Occasionally medical treatment was made conditional upon listening to sermons and the study of the New Testament.[11]

Medical Introduction

Palestine, which once experienced a glorious era of medical progress, had descended to its unprecedented nadir in this field by the end of the eighteenth century. The main reason for lowering the medical standards in the region, which forced the inhabitants of Palestine to rely mainly on folk medicine, was the prolonged and continuous decline of the Ottoman Empire. This deficiency in adequate medical services, which lasted until the mid-nineteenth century, was also the result of unsanitary conditions, poverty and ignorance, as well as a lack of public health facilities. This was manifested by sewage flowing through the streets, excessive garbage deposits, water drawn from untreated wells, overcrowded and unventilated quarters, and disregard for personal hygiene. These harsh conditions caused infectious diseases, and plagues broke out claiming many victims.[12]

The ancient sewerage system of Jerusalem was not working in the eighteenth and nineteenth century, according to Charles William Wilson (1835-1905) and Charles Warren (1840-1927). They penetrated the system while excavating in the city, and found out that the lines were blocked with rubbish. Eventually the mainline (230 metres long) that ended in Kidron Valley, was operational only after severe rain.[13] In 1863, British civil engineer John Irvine Whitty (b. 1822), a Fellow of the Royal Geographical Society of London, produced a book entitled: 'Proposed water supply and sewerage for Jerusalem: its present state and former resources'.[14]

The rubbish had built up for centuries, with piles of garbage to be found near the city walls and outside. These piles included stones, dust, ashes, rotten wood, animals' bones and organic matters. This was in addition to that found within the walls in the city streets. Some sources indicate that in many cases rubbish was thrown into low ancient rooms and when full, the rooms were sealed. In his report, Wilson described the accumulation of garbage, for instance, near the Armenian Garden, as piled 9 metres high, and near the city wall between Damascus and Lions gates being piled up to 20 metres high.[15] The sanitary condition deteriorated every year when thousands of pilgrims arrived in the city, with the lack of public toilets making it hard to be in town due to the bad smell.[16] Most of the nineteenth century sources report that the Jewish quarter was the unhealthiest place, due to the above mentioned conditions and the high density in which the Jewish inhabitants of the city lived.[17]

The most dangerous situation occurred after the winter rains when the increased flow of water would carry rubbish into the water cisterns and contaminate them. The vast majority of the inhabitants of the Holy City depended on water from cisterns since other means of water supply, such as pipes and ancient canals were either not working or did not exist.[18] The cisterns, already unclean, became filled with rubbish carried by the rainwater. In addition, very few inhabitants regularly cleaned their roofs, water canal and cisterns, remembering to let the first running water clean out the system and only then, to fill up the reservoirs. Whoever did this could get a good quality water, sometimes even better than the water that came through ancient un-cleaned pipes.

Titus Tobler (1806-1877), was a Swiss physician and researcher of Palestine who made four visits to the Holy Land (1835, 1845-6, 1857, 1865), each of which yielded articles and books reporting his research and his intellectual experiences. Tobler refers to that matter by writing that the cistern and the water pool were two of the main causes for the unhealthy conditions in Jerusalem. He determined that the vapour rising from them and the beverages made from their water caused diseases, even if they were cleaned frequently. He believed that vapour caused diseases, a common mistake before microbes were discovered. Tobler mentions the tanneries that operated within the city and the sewage, which was haphazard and very rarely processed, as other sources of disease.

The final cause he lists is the piles of rubbish, which had accumulated in houses, streets and outside the city walls.[19]

The lack of personal hygiene, which was a significant factor in the wretched medical conditions in Jerusalem, characterised all classes of the inhabitants of the city. There was, for example, a strong prejudice against washing children. The head of the English mission hospital described this attitude towards personal hygiene among the people of Jerusalem:

> They have a notion that a clean skin induces delicacy of constitution, and that dirt is the best preventive of diseases. Hence, even the children of the well-to-do people are often to be seen literally coated with a layer of filth and effete cuticle. Whether dirt, scanty diet, and foul air can of themselves produce fever is a question which is not necessary to discuss here.[20]

The many epidemics that spread in the city were described by almost every traveller and visitor; a sure sign of the presence of an epidemic was when the various monasteries closed their doors to foreigners. In some cases the governor closed the city gates, and in others the monasteries and the government established quarantines.[21] Among the most frequent diseases were malaria, eye infection, headaches, and dysentery, besides other infectious maladies and contagious childhood illnesses. Among the plagues were cholera, bubonic plague, typhoid fever, smallpox, and meningitis.[22] Some evidence dating from that period actually blamed the health situation on the city climate, its drinking water and the inhabitant's food supply.[23] However, one solution for the needs of personal hygiene was in fact the public bathhouses (*Hamam*). Jerusalem in the seventeenth century had six bathhouses one of which was called the medical bathhouse (*al-Shifa*).[24]

The Jewish physicians and the medical staff in Franciscan institutions were educated in Italy and else where in Europe, and were the forerunners of European medicine in Jerusalem. European medicine was reflected in European medical literature utilized by the local physicians as well as in the names of diseases and medications in Spanish, Portuguese, Italian and Latin listed in local publications. The Franciscan dispensary in Jerusalem with its rich library, its medical staff and the variety of medications it stocked, also contributed to the introduction of European medicine.[25]

150 years before the visits of the first English Physicians in Jerusalem, Rabbi Rephael Mordekhai Malki (d. 1702), a physician who acquired his medical education in Italy, and served as a community physician in Palestine from 1667 until his death in 1702, offered the following description:

> A physician in Jerusalem is hard to find, a knowledgeable one you cannot find at all, others that are not learned and knowledgeable are everywhere. This is because the medical knowledge of the eastern countries, the Turkish Empire… is poor… This is why it is impossible to be a physician in Jerusalem – its inhabitants and its scholars do not believe in real medicine and its practice. In their eyes, anyone who claims to be a doctor and a real physician are equal… In these circumstances, and considering the level of the physicians in the city, one must not turn to any of the doctors of Jerusalem, and whoever follows their instructions is a killer… Better that such doctors be absent than present, and rather… leave the sick in God's hand than place them in the hands of such a one.[26]

Of further interest is a description by the French traveller Comte Constantine François Volney (1757-1820) in the 1780s. After his visit to Jerusalem in 1785, Volney drew a gloomy picture of the condition of formal scientific knowledge in Syria and Egypt:

> If one were under pressure he might find a man knowledgeable enough to let blood and having the proper instrument to open a blood vessel. Once a doctor had ordered burn treatment, or written a simple recipe, he considered his work finished. That might be the reason that they ask for medical advice from every European servant, as if he were Esclapios in person. From where would learned physicians evolve if there were not the proper institutions?[27]

Conrad Schick (1822-1901), a German architect and researcher of Jerusalem who spent more than fifty years in that city, from 1846, has well described the medical situation in Palestine and Jerusalem.[28] Towards the end of the nineteenth century Schick wrote:

> Philanthropic organizations and wealthy individuals who had an interest in the Holy Land … can function in various spheres in Palestine: there is a lack of hospitals, qualified and experienced physicians and pharmacists in cities and in large population centres such as Hebron, Gaza, Shechem, Jenin, Tiberias, Safed, etc. It is necessary to promote the construction of hospitals and clinics staffed by young doctors. It is very important to set up a central institution or hospital and clinic for eye-disease patients in the centre of the country – preferably in Jerusalem.[29]

In the prolonged absence of sufficient medical care over a period of several generations, the outbreak of diseases and plagues was seen as a combination of inevitable fate and a heavenly decree. Over time, a variety of popular folk remedies was developed, based on old medical treatises and substances used in ancient times. Alongside these came cures, charms, amulets, incantations, and superstitions. These curative methods were often applied with the assistance of minor religious functionaries of all three faiths reciting passages from their scriptures and sending their flock to prostrate themselves on the graves of forefathers and saints buried in the Holy Land. The use of amulets and curative remedies was a common solution for incurable diseases, mainly mental illnesses. The terrible symptoms that accompanied such illnesses led those in contact with the patient to believe that magical powers and demons caused them, and that magical cures would therefore relieve the distress.

As an example of that kind of magical cure and superstition, one may mention the cure called then 'Indulco' or 'Indulca' (the word Indulca is most probably from the Latin 'Indulco' – to sweeten). This cure was used by the Spanish Jews for special diseases, such as madness, sudden blindness, sudden frights, epilepsy and barrenness. The treatment was divided into two classes, viz., the great and the small Indulca. A booklet published by the London Jews Society at the end of the 19 Century provided the following description:

The small Indulca – All the household of the patient, as well as all the neighbors who lived in the same enclosure or adjoining rooms, were obliged to leave their dwellings for a few days, and the patient was left alone in the chamber with a witch who was familiar with the secret. The said chamber had been previously emptied, whitewashed, washed, cleaned and all Holy Books removed. On the night when the Indulca was to be administered the patient was forbidden to pray, to recite the daily portion of Scripture, to mention the word heaven or anything concerning Holy Writ. The witch prepared a little wheat, barley, salt, water, milk, honey, four or six eggs, and sweetmeats or sugar. At midnight the witch mixed all these ingredients together and scattered a little round the sick bed, on the threshold, and in the four corners of the room, reciting meanwhile the following in a whisper:

> My Lords, I beseech you to pity, compassionate, and have mercy upon the soul (or life) of your servant, the patient (giving the name), the son or daughter of your maid (giving the mother's name), and overlook his or her trespasses; and if he or she have sinned and done any evil to you, forgive and pardon his or her sin; give his, or her life, and restore his or her health and strength, open her womb and loosen her bonds (if to those who lose their young children), give life to her sons and daughters, and let this honey and sugar be to sweeten your palates and mouths, the wheat and barley to feed your cattle and sheep, and the water and salt to establish peace, friendship, love and brotherhood, an everlasting covenant of salt between us and you.

At this stage the witch breaks the eggs and pours the same in the aforementioned places, kneels and prostrates herself, kisses the ground several times, and proceed with the following prayer: 'Here I offer to you life for life, in order that you may restore the life of this patient' (or his reason or whatever the case may be).

This was continued and repeated for two or more successive nights; and if the patient was not benefited it was continued seven or nine nights altogether. If the patient was poor and could not afford the requisite expenses, or if the neighbors declined to leave the adjoining rooms, then the witch went to either a cistern or bath, and there poured a little salt and water, and prayed as before and said 'Behold! Water and salt to be a covenant of peace between us'.

The great Indulca - differs from the former only in being prolonged for 45 nights, the patient being required to dress in rich white garments, and the room, in addition to the aforesaid cleansing etc., to be well lit with many wax candles, and besides the aforementioned ingredients, there must be various savoury dishes and spices, and the aforementioned witchcraft was continued.[30]

Folk medicine of this type, which is common in most cultures of the world, began to lose its standing in Europe with the development of modern medicine. Among the inhabitants of the Near East its use was still deeply rooted during the late nineteenth century and even into the twentieth century. Such cures are characteristic of a few countries in the world even today, and some of their components can be found in popular folk remedies among various Jewish communities and minority groups in Israel.

The Swiss physician Titus Tobler reported that traditional medicine was very common among all the inhabitants of Jerusalem, without any ethnic or religious differences.[31] Only a few learned physicians lived in the city, and many among the local people preferred to get medical help from different kinds of healers.[32] He describes his meetings with many healers of different skills and faiths, Jews, Christians, and Muslims. He censured treatment administered by an old Jewish woman, which, he wrote, 'created major damage, especially in the treatment of eye inflammations'. Another method of treatment that was very popular, according to Tobler, was bloodletting. He reported that Jewish, Christian, and Muslim men were in the practice of opening blood vessels with a wide variety of contrivances and special instruments. In the past they had performed this treatment on the streets, but later it was practiced indoors. It was done gratis for the poor and at a small fee for the rest of the patients. Tobler refuted the common belief of Muslim objection to bloodletting, which, he asserted, his own experience proved unfounded.[33]

Barbers too engaged in 'bloodletting', or more accurately 'blood sucking'. Tobler describes several Arab barbers and one Jewish, who practiced a different method of blood release. They scratched the skin, placed the base of an animal's horn over the wound, and sucked the blood from the cut top of the horn. That way they did not touch the blood. The suction continued for about thirty minutes, and the barbers used a piece of leather to preserve the vacuum pressure when they had to breathe. 'This method, which is well known all over the East, was once common in our land [Switzerland] and is still in practice in some spa sites'. The scratching and sucking was done on the arms and the neck. The use of a cupping glass for blood letting was reported as well.[34]

The level of medicine can be measured according to a number of criteria. The main ones are a standarized system of public health, formal medical training, and proven medicinal substances. Medical science in Palestine in general and Jerusalem in particular exemplified the continuation of classical Hippocratic-Galenic medical methods adopted and improved by the Muslims in the course of the Middle Ages. In the regions under Turkish rule, important centres were set up in which physicians of repute were engaged in the art of healing, research, writing and teaching. During the eighteenth and the first half of the nineteenth century, Palestine and the outlying areas lacked such centres where prominent physicians could practice medicine, so that this region did not produce any trained medical practitioners.

Throughout most of the Ottoman period, Palestine was considered an area of marginal importance. It was far from the centres of culture and government, and eminent physicians avoided going there. The situation portrayed in the preceding chapter gives a general view of medical realities during that period. However, the practice of medicine in Jerusalem should be examined in greater detail since it was made up of three main strata: public medicine, communal medicine, and private medicine. A fourth stratum, voluntary medicine, gained ground only in the course of the nineteenth century, and will be addressed below.

Public Medicine

Jerusalem, like other large cities of the Ottoman Empire, offered minimal access to medical services. These services were meant to supply the needs of the general population without prejudice of religion or nationality; however, by the discriminating nature of the local regime, it was only the Arab population that benefited from these services. The function of the general public hospital in Jerusalem, which operated throughout the Ottoman period, was the continuation of a medical institution dating from the time of the Ayyubid Caliphate of the twelfth and thirteenth centuries. The institution had different sections: a general hospital, a hospital for the mentally ill, and an eye clinic. Physicians who served at this hospital, which was also supported by the central government, received official appointments from the government, providing a salary and premiums. These physicians were not allowed to leave the city without stating a good reason, obtaining a permit, and finding a replacement. The physical condition of the general public hospital deteriorated in time, and despite all attempts to repair it, the building remained partially in ruins. The standard of this institution, like that of similar institutions, deteriorated parallel with the inexorable decline of the Ottoman Empire itself.[35]

Only in 1886 did the Jerusalem Municipality establish a clinic, but even that functioned only three days a week. In 1891, the Municipal Hospital was erected in Sheikh Bader (today 86 Jaffa Street, in the heart of Jerusalem, to be dealt later on page 156).[36] The inhabitants of Jerusalem were therefore limited to the medicinal substances in use throughout the region for centuries. As time passed, the variety of medications decreased because of disruptions in the trade routes. In addition, harsh economic conditions halted the demand for exotic and expensive substances, and there was a lowering of standards among physicians and care givers.[37] Out of the scores of substances mentioned in the various historical sources on the medical situation in Jerusalem until the beginning of the nineteenth century, only quinine is listed as a medicinal compound introduced from the new world of modern medicine. This medication was prescribed in the dispensaries of the Franciscan community in Jerusalem during the first half of the eighteenth century.[38]

In that same century, new medicinal substances from Africa, Asia, and America were important components in the reservoir of medications, as attested in the volumes of *materia medica*[39] By contrast, in Jerusalem and elsewhere in Palestine, the greater number of medicinal substances used by authorized physicians were traditional. As indicated by their plant, mineral, and animal origins, these were derived mostly from local sources in the period under discussion.[40]

Communal Medicine

Communal medicine, which gained adherents in Jerusalem, was an essential service of the various ethnic groups in order to provide an alternative to the defective public health system. For religious reasons, Jews and Christians, with the permission of the Ottoman government, preferred to use the advanced medical services of their own communities. However, in all probability, there also existed local Muslim almshouses, offering limited medical care as well.[41]

The centre of communal medicine for the Jews of Jerusalem from the sixteenth to the eighteenth century was their own hospital located in the Jewish Quarter. This hospital apparently belonged to the Oriental Jewish (*Sephardi*) community, while the European Jewish (*Ashkenazi*) community, which was recognized as a separate minority group, sometimes operated its own hospital.[42] A reliable description of the Jewish hospital, which was called Bikkur Holim, can be found in the writings of the physician Rabbi Rephael Mordekhai Malki. From his description it appears that the hospital was headed by the community treasurer, who, in the absence of a physician, was the supreme medical authority. The institution was supported mainly through contributions from the Jewish community in Amsterdam, and with these funds the treasurer bought food and medicine for the patients. One of his main duties was to prepare a drink containing sugar, almonds, and rosewater, mixed with various condiments as could be afforded, and to distribute the drink to patients in their homes.[43]

An important factor that contributed to the introduction of European medicine in the Holy Land was the Franciscan activity, conducted in Acre, Nazareth, Bethlehem, and especially Jerusalem. The seventeenth and eighteenth centuries were the height of the operation of the Franciscan medical center in Jerusalem. The medical centre was in decline at the nineteenth century, but lasted until the twentieth century.[44] The monastery had at its disposal a library containing a wealth of professional medical literature of the European school.[45] They applied new techniques in medicine in general, and military medicine in particular, but this had no immediate effect on the state of medicine in Jerusalem.[46]

Evidence of the flourishing of the Franciscan Medical Center in Jerusalem in the seventeenth and the eighteenth centuries, is the variety of medications from all over the world that were available there, a staff of certified pharmacists trained in Europe and modern medical equipment. Since there was no other pharmacy in Jerusalem, this one served people of all Christian denominations and distributed medicines free of charge.[47]

The Franciscans did not practice medicine in Europe, but while they were stationed in Jerusalem they had no alternative but to provide medical care for Catholic pilgrims to the Holy Land. At first, they sent monks who were qualified as physicians, pharmacists, surgeons, and nurses to Jerusalem. Most were from Italy, and only a few arrived from other European countries such as France and Spain.[48] In addition, a large number of medical practitioners, nurses, pharmacists, physicians, and even surgeons served in the Franciscan medical institutions in Jerusalem until the nineteenth century, most of them having been sent from Italy whither they returned at the end of their period of service. The patients were treated and hospitalized in the boarding house for the poor, located in the Christian quarter of the Old City, separate from the monastery.

T he dispensary developed rapidly into one of the largest of its kind in the East. It contained a wide variety of medications and was run by a staff trained in modern European institutions.[49] The dispensary became famous for its innovative medicines, especially for the 'Jerusalem Balsam' mixed by secret formula and containing forty different medicinal ingredients. An impressive medical library and a spacious, modern European-style pharmacy were at the disposal of the medical staff.

A reliable description of the contents of the dispensary at the beginning of the eighteenth century is given by Elzar Horn, a

Franciscan monk of German origin who resided in the Holy Land from 1724 to 1744:

> The dispensary in Jerusalem is one of the best in the Christian world. The storehouses contain medications of all kinds which were purchased with donated funds, and especially with funds contributed for this specific purpose by the Venetian Republic.[50]

The Swedish botanist Frederick Hasselquist (1722-1752), who visited the institution in 1750, reported,

> It was amazing to see the quantities of expensive medications stored there. … Here they prepare the Jerusalem Balsam so famed in these countries … it is very effective for all fresh external wounds. … The whole pharmacopoeia (dispensary stock) is valued at several hundred thousand piasters.[51]

In 1806 the German traveller, Jasper Ulrich Seetzen (1767-1811), was impressed by the pharmacy, which was the biggest he saw in the East. He wrote about the monks' garden, where medicinal plants were cultivated, and noted that he received 'two bottles of real Balsam with written indications of its qualities'.[52]

Francisco Lopez, a Spanish friar, was a physician and pharmacist who practiced in Jerusalem between 1788 and 1813. Another friar who worked as a physician was Joaqim Martinez (1800-1873), who practiced medicine and was a pharmacist in Jerusalem for 47 years (1826-1873). A third friar who worked in nineteenth century Palestine was Giovanni da Trieste (1806-1874), who practiced medicine in Jerusalem (1842-1852) and Bethlehem (1854-1862).[53] Their influence on Jerusalem society was limited, since they did not treat the needy social economic strata, e.g. the poor Muslims and Jews. Travellers and other patients reported that they were good physicians. It seems that both the institution and the practitioners supplied medical treatment, mainly to members of the local Catholic community, travellers, and sometimes to other Christians and even in special cases treated prominent Muslims (Jazzar Pasha, Governor of Acre in 1775-1804)[54] and Jews (Hayim David Hazan

(1790-1869) the *Hacham Bashi* (*Sephardic* Chief Rabbi) of Jerusalem in 1861-1869).[55]

Not much is known about the friars' medical education; however, after serving so many years in Jerusalem it seems unlikely that they were well informed about medical developments occurring elsewhere.

Moreover, since the monastery and its medical institution were attached mainly to Spain and Italy, which did not lead the field with respect to physicians and medicine in Europe during that period, the Franciscans' importance declined immensely. They could not compete with the medical institutions and practitioners sent from European imperialists powers such as England, France, Germany, and Russia to Jerusalem in the second half of the nineteenth century.[56]

Private Medicine

A small number of patients in Jerusalem preferred to use the services of private physicians, who received them in clinics generally set up in rented shops in the city quarters. During the seventeenth and eighteenth centuries a few Muslim and Jewish physicians served in a private capacity, most of them being public physicians who engaged in private medicine in their spare time. The title of physician in this period needs explanation, since generally, there were two types of physicians in Palestine and Jerusalem. One type were popular physicians without professional training in a medical institution. These included eye healers, who were not mentioned in government listings so they worked with the semi-official permission of the authorities. The other type was qualified physicians, who were professionally trained at a hospital or other medical institution, or who were accredited by well-known physicians. The qualified physicians arriving from Europe, Christians and Jews alike, had received their training at various Universities, especially in Italy. All qualified physicians received written authorization from the institution where they had studied or from the government, with explicit indication as to the area of their specialization. The physicians in Jerusalem were members of a professional association headed by the Chief Physician of

Jerusalem, who was charged by the government with supervising medical standards and professional training.[57]

Pharmacies

Pharmacies in Jerusalem, and to latter extent elsewhere in Palestine, produced, imported and distributed various medicinal substances and drugs. Key testimony to this phenomenon is found in the writings of Titus Tobler.[58] Following his long journey to Palestine (one of several) in the winter of 1845-46, he wrote the book *Beitrage zur Medizinischen Topographie von Jerusalem* (A description of medical conditions in Jerusalem),[59] in which he drew a unique picture of that aspect of life. According to his observations, there were four European pharmacies functioning in Jerusalem in 1846: the Franciscan pharmacy, the best known in the city, was located in the Franciscan monastery. Being the longest standing European pharmacy in Jerusalem, it was highly thought of through the ages. Tobler wrote in his notebook, after visiting the pharmacy:

> The place looks ancient... the laboratory is strange, unmatched by any European competitor for being so strange... the instruments have old-fashioned shapes, like the traditional tools of mystic alchemy and astrology.... Together with those instruments were some skeletons, surgical instruments, threatening monsters covered with mould... different type of amulets... and all in ancient dark rooms. Yet the store room of the medicinal substances was exceptionally fine.

The Greek Orthodox pharmacy, according to Tobler was '[t]he cleanest of all, it was bright and well designed. The names of medicines were written in magnificent Greek lettering. The Greek Orthodox inhabitants and pilgrims received the medication free of charge'.[60] The Jewish pharmacy was located in Dr Shimon Fränkel's house. Fränkel (1806-1880), a Jewish physician of German origin, was sent in 1843 by Sir Moses Montefiore (1784-1885), the British Jewish philanthropist, to establish a Jewish hospital in the holy city.[61] Tobler recalled some medicine sellers whose 'pharmacies' were in the Jewish quarter and were better equipped than those of the Arab drug sellers. Two of these were 'of importance; the names of the medicines were written in Hebrew and cleanliness was non-existent'. Tobler added that he found there the 'Kalomel' and an opium concoction that he could not find in the Arab drug market. He also found theriac and other materials. He concluded this subject thus: 'Other than at the Christian pharmacies, physicians could find the most essential substances here, as long as they could read the drug's [Hebrew] name'.[62]

Tobler gives an exceptional account of a visit to *Suk al-Attarin*, the drug market of Jerusalem in the north-west of the city. He made a list of the substances he saw in one shop, which is probably the only list of medicinal substances in Jerusalem ever published. It was written as a distorted transliteration in German script of the Arabic names, and it subsequently has been translated and studied. It contains 81 substances and is similar to lists drawn up in the same market at the end of the 20th century.[63]

Tobler's observations in his book *Beitrage zur medizinischen Topographie von Jerusalem* are the best source for a discussion of the common illness and diseases in Palestine.[64] Nevertheless, one should note that his interpretation of the particular disease and illness cannot always be credited with real or modern meanings. He wrote in the 1850s, before the 'Laboratory Revolution' and the modern medical paradigm, namely germ theory.[65]

Common diseases and epidemics

(arranged in alphabetical order)

Burns: 'very frequent, mainly among children, due to the common use of the mangals (griddles)'.[66]

Cataract 'is widespread in Jerusalem, Dr. [Edward] Macgowan, [1795-1860, the head of the English Mission Hospital in Jerusalem] informed me, and therefore encouraged the establishment of the Hospital... Though other physicians such as myself… agreed that cataract was rare in Jerusalem, and we had not heard about a surgery performed in the last 15 months since the hospital was established'.[67] Nevertheless, before his arrival in the city, he states that British surgeon had performed some successful surgery. In any case the inhabitants did not trust European eye medicine and preferred to use common powder (unrecognized).

Cholera: 'this disease exists in the Holy Land and Jerusalem'.[68]

Constipation: 'observed frequently, especially when connected with haemorrhoids'.[69]
Diarrhoea: 'plentiful, all year around, and sometimes evolved into dysentery'. The hot climate and high consumption of fruits such as almonds, apricots, and oranges were believed to be the cause. Tobler mentions his personal experiences of diarrhoea.[70]
Dysentery: 'common especially in the summer when the figs and grapes are ripe'. Usually the disease was not deadly, but every once in a while it was accompanied with high temperature. The usual treatment was theriac.[71]
Erysipelas: 'widespread', and was treated with a wide variety of cures including red earth with human urine or silk threads.[72]
High temperature: 'very common', acute temperature necessitating treatment. A sugar water drink was administered to fight the thirst as a long-standing Arab remedy.[73]
Hysteria: 'frequent'.[74]
Inflammations and haemorrhages: 'frequent'.[75]
Iritis and keratitis: 'very frequent diseases, mainly among children. Most of the cases are chronic'. Tobler describes shocking cases, aggravated by 'wrong' treatment with irritating substances of the 'healer' women. Inflammations and swellings were very common and many blind people were to be found on the streets.[76]
Laryngitis and cold: 'widespread all year round, mainly after the first winter rain and especially when cold easterly winds blow'.[77]
Malaria: 'one of the most common diseases in the city'. The European physicians agreed that it appeared frequently all year round, but reached a peak in the spring. The disease struck everyone, including babies and nursing mothers. The fever appeared in its single, double, triple, and even quadruple form. The high temperature was not fatal. Tobler seeks its cause in the 'consumption of uncooked fruits', and has heard that it 'might be from poisonous vapour coming from the Dead Sea', A likely cause, he indicates, could well be the water kept in the dirty cisterns and pools. Dr Edward Macgowan asserted that dwelling near the Patriarch pool was unhealthy and vulnerable to malaria. Tobler conducted a study and concluded that 'there were a considerable number of cases of malaria near the pool, more than in other parts of the city'. He blames the vapour and not the quality of the

drinking water. The high temperature was treated with large quantities of quinine (Tobler was critical of the quantities). The inhabitants used a 'traditional medication', which consisted of: 'apricot seeds, aniseed, rue, lemon juice and urine. They also used amulets, a vegetarian diet for 40 days and other magics'.[78]

Oriental leprosy: 'Leprosy is a common disease in the East, and Jerusalem hosts many lepers, who dwell in their separate huts near Zion Gate'. Tobler describes the symptoms and progress of the disease: 'I saw men without beards.... People without teeth...and patients without fingers...the urine is yellow and the excrement is black'. Death from this terrible disease was sudden. Tobler informs us its cause was unknown, and that it was a genetic condition (an early and unique remark for the mid-nineteenth century, but erroneous). Although there was no cure, Tobler lists some treatments: bloodletting, leeches, purgatives, bath, fast, magic, and use of substances such as mercury and snakes. He concludes this unpleasant subject on a humanitarian note. How is it, he wonders, that 'the British, who show overdone sympathy towards the Jews, are apathetic to this disaster.... A human, compassionate heart would have found the way to get them back to human society. Humanity has many means to fight leprosy'.[79]

Oriental Plague and Smallpox: 'It did not cross my mind to describe perfectly this affliction of Jerusalem'. But Tobler does try to describe the disease and to convey as much information as he can. 'First cases are very hard to diagnose – even for an experienced physician, though after a while anyone could recognize the disease'. Tobler admitted that very little was known about the disease and that no empirical proof existed for the notion that the plague evolved from the smell of decayed human bodies. However, he concurred with the idea that the bad smell of bodies and rotten garbage in the streets encouraged the progress of the plague. In addition, 'somewhere, somehow the disease is self-generating'. Tobler describes some experiments conducted by the Russian and the Ottoman authorities to learn the cause of the disease. 'The best solution is isolation', he writes, which the Latin monastery practiced in cases of plague. Tobler reports that the plague had struck the country in 1801, 1812, 1834, 1838-9, and 1840-1. He concludes his report, 'as far as I could find the plague always hit Jerusalem in the hot season, especially spring and summer'.[80]

Pneumonia: 'appears frequently, in all seasons. Accompanied by high temperature. Dr. Fraenkel cured it with bloodletting and alkali with saltpetre'.[81]

Rheumatism: 'common disease, all year round, less in summer. Sometimes accompanied by high temperature. The disease usually causes pain in the chest and the neck'.[82]

Stomach diseases: 'common and followed by high temperature'. 'They are caused by uncooked food, gourmandising on sweets, coffee drinking, smoking and early sexual satisfaction'.[83] The common treatment was purgatives and induced vomiting.

Tetanus: 'Dr. Fraenkel observed it frequently among children… Dr. Assuani reported only one case…'.[84]

Tonsillitis: 'widespread, especially among children, accompanied by coughing. According to Dr. Fraenkel's experience the disease was not deadly and the patient could recover without bloodletting'. Tobler adds a personal observation: he suffered from tonsillitis himself, was troubled by it for some days and then enjoyed a full recovery.[85]

Wounds: 'were hardly seen by Dr. Fraenkel, who added that they become cured quickly'.[86]

Rare diseases

Asthma: 'rare disease'.[87] However, Tobler's conclusion is strange in light of the many medieval sources relating that asthma was a common disease in the Levant.[88]

Chickenpox: 'rare in Jerusalem. Had never been seen by Dr. Fraenkel'.[89]

Coughing: 'rare, appeared in intensified form among children'.[90]

Enteritis: 'a rare disease', and according to Tobler treated wrongly by the local physician.[91]

Loss of voice: 'rare, Dr. Fraenkel reported only two cases'.

Migraine: 'rare'.[92]

Pleurisy: 'was observed rarely by both Dr. Fraenkel and Dr. Assuani'.[93]

Psychotic disorders: 'rare, if we do not count stupidity as such a disease', writes Tobler: 'patients do not seek help from a physician,

but from religious authorities such as Muslim sheikhs or monks in a monastery'. Tobler states that there was no suicide.[94]
Epidemics Typhus: 'rare disease; neither Dr. Fraenkel nor Dr. Assuani had seen a case in three years'.
Rabies: 'was observed neither in Jerusalem nor in any other city in the East'.[95]

ENGLISH MISSION HOSPITALS

Early Attempts by Medical Missionaries in Jerusalem

In the framework of unsuccessful exploratory tours conducted by some missionaries in the Land of Israel, beginning in 1820, the British missionary William Bucknor Lewis spent a brief period of time in the country.[1] In May 1824, Lewis sent a detailed report to London from his home base in Beirut on the situation of the Jews in Palestine, in which he recommended ways of increasing the chances of success for future emissaries. Lewis proposed that the Jews should not be treated as a homogenous group but that one should distinguish between the two main communities. In his opinion, missionaries of German origin should be sent to act within the German-speaking *Ashkenazi* community and at the same time British missionaries should be sent to work among the *Sephardi* communities. As for the location of the permanent mission stations, Lewis reported that the Jews lived in four cities – Jerusalem, Hebron, Safed and Tiberias. Therefore, at this stage, two stations should be set up: one in Jerusalem that would cover the activities in Hebron, and the other in Safed that would include the Jewish community in Tiberias. At the end of his report, Lewis warned that the mission should not expect openness from the local Jews towards the Christian faith unless they were prepared to die as martyrs, to escape from the country, or to find someone to protect them.[2]

About one month after Lewis sent the summary of his visit to the Land of Israel and his proposals with regard to the manner in which a permanent mission should be founded, the non-Jewish

London Jews Society sent George Edward Dalton (d. 1826), as its missionary to Jerusalem. Dalton, a native of Wexford in Ireland and a doctor by profession, was sent to provide an additional dimension to the work of the mission.[3] In this way the London Jews Society came close to being a pioneer in the field of medical missions in the Land of Israel. In June 1824, Dalton left with his family for Malta, where his wife gave birth to a son. After a stay of a few months, the family sailed to Alexandria, and on January 6, 1825 they landed in Beirut and took up residence in temporary lodgings prepared for them by William Lewis. Dalton's departure for Jerusalem was postponed because of the illness of his son, and he was forced to remain in Beirut until the end of March. Only then he set out, and chose the route that passed through Acre, Nazareth, the Jezreel Valley and Shechem. On April 2, 1825, Dalton entered the Damascus Gate in Jerusalem and met his colleague Lewis.[4]

A few days after Dalton's arrival, he and Lewis were caught in the throes of riots resulting from the rebellion against sharp tax increases imposed by the Governor of Damascus who was responsible for the Land of Israel as well.[5] During the riots, the Governor's soldiers rampaged against the non-Muslim and foreign community in Jerusalem following allegations of property thefts from Muslims in Bethlehem by Greek Orthodox monks from the Monastery of Mar Elias. The two missionaries took part in calming the atmosphere, with Dalton treating the injured and Lewis obtaining the release of one of the rabbis who had been arrested.[6] By mid-May, the gloomy effect that these events left upon these two men raised apprehensions concerning the difficulties to be expected in setting up a permanent mission in the city. Dalton reported at that time that there was a prohibition against the distribution of the Holy Scriptures and on the problems of full range missionary work, but he found a small ray of hope in his contacts with the rabbis of Jerusalem. In his opinion, the Jews of the Land of Israel valued the English nation very highly, and for that reason the sting was taken out of the Jews' traditional bias against the Christians. It seems that the comradely relationship Dalton and Lewis developed with the rabbis was earned by the medical assistance that they had provided.

Already towards the middle of April 1825, the disquiet increased in Jerusalem. Most of the foreigners began to organize an escape from the city. Only at the beginning of May were the missionaries told that they were permitted to leave Jerusalem for Beirut. Dalton and his family spent most of the summer in Beirut in anticipation of a permit that would allow him to take up permanent residence in Jerusalem. However, his health began to deteriorate and the family preferred to transfer to the city of Tyre where his second son was born. They spent the autumn of 1825 in Tyre, waiting for news that the riots in Jerusalem had abated. In the meantime, Dalton planned an alternative journey to Safed, but was unable to travel because of his bad health. At the beginning of the winter, British travellers brought glad tidings from Jerusalem that calm was being restored in the city. Dalton decided to go there on his own for an extensive visit of three months, and for that purpose he transferred his family from Tyre back to Beirut. He departed in mid-December 1825 and on Christmas Day he reached Jerusalem and went to live among his Greek Orthodox friends.[7]

Dalton was joined in Jerusalem by John Nicolayson, the prominent figure of the London Jews Society in the Land of Israel.[8] On January 5, 1826 in spite of Dalton's indisposition, they set forth to visit the nearby city of Bethlehem. As soon as they arrived, Dalton again fell ill. Three days later the two men retraced their journey to the Greek Orthodox monastery in Jerusalem, and Dalton's health continued to deteriorate. On his deathbed Dalton managed to write the following:

> I feel as one dying… Tell the committee that the friends of the cause in England have too high an opinion of what has been done here, for as to the establishing of a mission in Jerusalem, or any other place in the country, nothing has been done as yet.[9]

On January 25, 1826, he succumbed to his illness and was buried at his own request in the Greek cemetery on Mount Zion.[10]

Dalton's stay in Palestine was very brief and he did not manage to leave his mark as a physician. But he was warmly welcomed by the inhabitants of Jerusalem even though he was an active missionary, and for that reason was important to the development of British medicine in the Land of Israel in years to come. After Dalton's death, the following words were written in the bulletin of the London Jews Society:

> Dr Dalton seemed to be a man peculiarly well suited to the sphere in which he was called to labour. His amiable manners, his undissembled piety, and his medical skill, had all united to gain him the esteem and attention of the inhabitants of Palestine. While, however, we were anticipating much good, under the divine blessing, from his patients and preserving labours in the earthly Canaan, it has pleased the Lord to call him to a heavenly one, and it becomes us to bow in humble submission assured that 'He doeth all things well'.[11]

With Dalton's death, the attempt to engage in medical practice within the framework of the mission activities was broken off for a decade. Nicolayson, the representative of the London Jews Society in Jerusalem, was also forced to leave Palestine a year after Dalton's death. This was for reasons of regional politics that led in 1831 to a war that raged in the country between Egypt and the Ottoman Empire. Only in 1833, after the Egyptian conquest and the establishment of Egyptian rule, which brought a tolerant attitude towards foreigners, did Nicolayson return to set up the mission station in Jerusalem.

In December 1838, the medical activities of the London Jews Society in Jerusalem were reactivated with the arrival of two missionaries who were Jewish converts. One of them was Albert Wilhelm Gerstmann (1815-1841), a doctor by profession who had received two years of training in Berlin and one year in London. With him came his chemist assistant, Melville Peter Bergheim (1815-1890). The two men stayed for a while in Beirut on their way to Jerusalem. Nicolayson repeatedly urged them, in a series of letters, to hasten their arrival, in order to help in the struggle against the plague that had begun to spread in Jerusalem in the spring of 1838.[12]

Gerstmann and his medical skills introduced a new dimension to the work of the Jerusalem mission. The leaders of the London Jews Society viewed his activities as of the greatest importance and defined his tasks one by one:

> You are further directed to attend as a Medical Capacity first of all **gratis** [original emphasis] to all who are connected to the Mission, & also to the poor Jews who may apply for advice or medicines [...from] Jews or others who can afford to pay you are allowed to take a reasonable fee.[13]

Gerstmann arrived in Jerusalem at the height of the plague and found that besides the miserable state of health among the Jews in the city because of poor conditions, their situation was even worse because of the inadequate medical care they received from Isaac Russhee, the local Jewish healer. In May 1839, Gerstmann requested the help of the British Consul to stop Russhee, a native Jerusalemite who engaged in medicine but had caused damage that led to the death of more people than those who had died of the plague itself. Gerstmann also asserted that Jerusalem would not be cured of the illness so long as people like Russhee were allowed to engage in medical practices.[14]

Members of the Jewish community, including a few rabbis, were grateful to Gerstmann and even began to show interest in the possibility of conversion to Christianity. Nicolayson, who was surprised by the extent of this phenomenon, wrote an emotional letter to Alexander McCaul (1799-1863), the Irish missionary and a prominent activist in the London Jews Society since its foundation.[15] In his letter, Nicolayson expressed for the first time his sense of the immense importance that should be given to medical activity as a major component in the success of missionary work.[16] He therefore laid before McCaul his plans and the need to raise funds among supporters of the London Jews Society for this purpose:

> Our plan is to form something that may grow into a hospital. For this purpose we need one who will become the advocate of Jewish misery in happy England, present the claims of Abraham's descendants in Jerusalem. ... Such (as said) **you** [original emphasis] either must become yourself, or find an equally suitable substitute. We can take no refusal, and offer you no other alternative. Yet be not alarmed at the name Hospital. We are not going to erect a place like the hospitals in London.[17]

This energetic appeal had its effect. At the first conference in which McCaul presented the new funding needs in Jerusalem, fifteen pounds sterling were collected.

The first blossoming of the Jerusalem Mission as a result of Gerstmann's medical success revealed a new need that had not so far been identified. The fact that a small group of Jews had joined the missionaries necessitated special evaluation and additional resources. In order to meet these needs, Nicolayson dispatched a letter similar in content to the one sent to McCaul, in which he requested immediate assistance from the leaders of the London Jews Society. He pointed out the urgent requirement of an additional building to house the clinic, pharmacy and a small storeroom for Gerstmann's medications. At the plenary session of the London Jews Society in March 1839, the members seriously considered the optimistic reports about additional Jews who had joined the circle of those interested in missionary work as a result of Gerstmann's medical successes, and also heard about the growing needs of the mission station for that reason. At this same session the London Jews Society adopted the decision to set up a temporary fund intended for immediate relief in Jerusalem.

In October 1839, as usually occurred in the autumn, the number of those stricken with disease reached its peak, and the limited medical services of the mission had to be activated in full force. Gerstmann worked day and night to preserve the health of the inhabitants in the city, and during that month he treated dozens of patients daily, which came to about 100 a day. Bergheim also joined in the task, and besides his work as a chemist he was also obliged to carry out purely medical procedures and simple surgery.[18] At the beginning of November, Gerstmann fell ill, lay close to death, and recovered with great difficulty. The Jews of Jerusalem in their gratitude towards him held a special prayer at the Western Wall for his recovery.

The dramatic rise in the medical activities with their accompanying missionary enterprise made it necessary to reassess the current circumstances. Nicolayson sent a request to the London Jews Society to set up a hospital in Jerusalem as soon as possible. The Society approved his request and established a fund to recruit the resources for this purpose, and even instructed Nicolayson to withdraw an initial sum of 100 pounds sterling.[19] Nicolayson took advantage of the fact that preparations were already under way to lay the foundations of other mission buildings, and he therefore gave instructions to renovate the roofs of the older buildings of the London Jews Society so as to install the Mission Hospital of Jerusalem in them. In January 1840, this ambitious project was frustrated. Gerstmann's long illness delayed the establishment of the hospital. And even after Gerstmann recovered, his weak condition made it necessary for him to return to England, and the hospital plans were postponed until a replacement could be found for him. In the meantime, the chemist Bergheim was put in charge of the medical wing of the mission, and was aided by the American physician, Cornelius Van-Dyck (1818-1895) who was then residing in Jerusalem. From August 1840, the London Jews Society began publishing a series of announcements in its bulletin seeking candidates capable of setting up a hospital in Jerusalem and managing the medical department. In March 1841, Nicolayson wrote with satisfaction that he was happy to hear a suitable candidate had been found.

First Hospital in Jerusalem

The modest medical services established by the London Jews Society in the late 1830s were abandoned during the second war between the Egyptians and the Ottoman Empire in 1840. But the Society knew that the work done by the missionary doctors had left an impression on the Jews of Jerusalem, and realized how essential the continuation of medical services was to achieving the society's goals. Its leaders were encouraged to give substance to their decision of March 1841 to renew their activities after the enforced interruption owing to the war. It was resolved to carry out the plans for founding a hospital for the Jews, and that next to it 'a School be established in Jerusalem under the immediate direction and management of the Head of the Medical department, and in which Surgery and Pharmacology is to be taught'. Also Dr Edward Macgowan was selected to serve as a doctor at the Jerusalem Mission.[20]

Macgowan arrived in Jerusalem in January 1842, and at the end of his first working month sent a detailed report describing the poor state of health of Jerusalem's Jews, and further describing his activities and his recommendations for the construction of a hospital and dispensary by the London Jews Society. He urged the London committee to reach some practical decision on this matter, and hinted that it would be possible to economize on the expenses of the medical department if the mission grew its own medicinal herbs. Macgowan even urged the Society to let him lease some land for this purpose and to employ a local gardener. While still awaiting permission from London, he began to renovate a small building for use as a dispensary to render first aid to Jewish patients and as a centre for the sale of medicines. Macgowan also conducted a few simple operations with the aid of equipment purchased in England.[21]

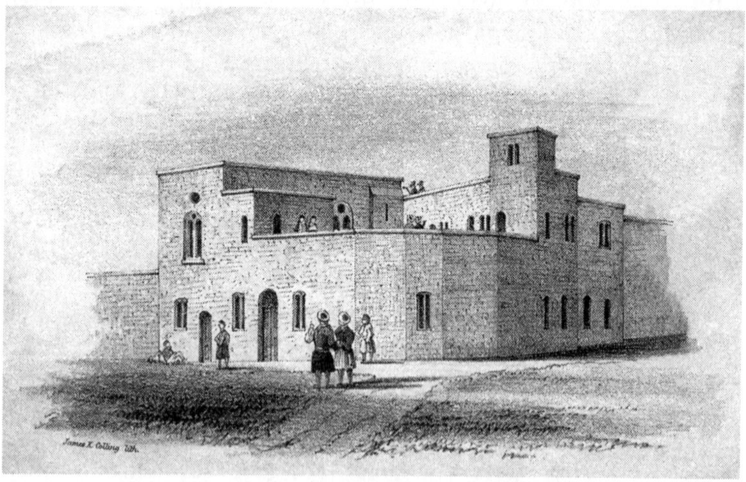

Figure 1, The first hospital within the city walls, Jerusalem

In mid-1842, Macgowan received permission from London to establish a modest hospital. He immediately set to work, and in September he managed to close an eleven-year lease on a building at £25 per annum. The building was near the Society's dispensary on the eastern slopes of Mount Zion facing the city, and near the Jewish Quarter. The hospital was planned to have twelve beds on two separate floors, the lower floor for men and the upper for women. At the same time, Macgowan proposed setting aside a separate wing for pilgrims and British tourists needing medical attention, and to charge fees to cover expenses and even to generate income.[22]

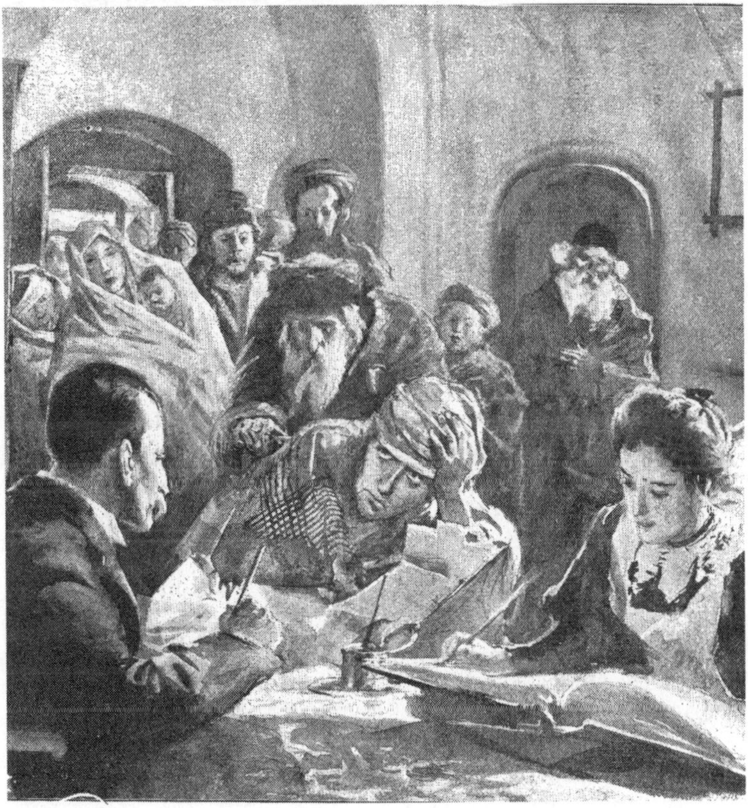

Figure 2 - The doctor and a nurse in the old hospital, Jerusalem

On December 12, 1844, the English Mission Hospital for the Jews was opened in Jerusalem, and within days was filled to capacity. The missionaries' frequent reports to London revealed their pride in their new hospital. The Society journal published many of Macgowan's letters, one of which described a typical day at the hospital:

> It has frequently been my wish during the last month, that our friends in England could get a peep at the hospital on one of my days for the admission of patients. The scene that would meet their eyes would be one of uncommon gratification and interest. They would see the waiting room full of patients, besides a crowd of others thronging the doors of the hospital, who had been too late for admission, but who are patiently waiting, in the hope of being attended to when the first applicants shall be dismissed. Every three or four minutes the door of the consultation-room opens, and out comes a patient with his prescription in his hand, which he takes to the dispensary, which is situated on the other side of the street. This lasts for about two hours, during which the crowd of patients in the street are waiting -- some standing, others seated, or lying on the ground or on the steps of the door. Some of them, naturally enough, lose patience, and, on the opening of the door, endeavour to force their way into the consulting-room, and are with difficulty prevented from doing so. Their turn, however, comes at last, when it becomes necessary to discriminate between those who really require advice, and those who are suffering from want. To the most necessitous of the latter a ticket is given for the matron of the hospital, who is in attendance in an adjoining room, and who, on receiving the ticket, gives out of her stores which have been provided by the kind friends in England, some articles of clothing, flour, or relief in a little money, according to the wants of the applicant.[23]

Jewish opposition to the Hospital

Even before the hospital's dedication ceremony and in spite of the three years' experience in operating the dispensary, the missionaries in Jerusalem anticipated opposition by the heads of the Jewish community to the hospitalization of Jewish patients in a Christian establishment. They tried to make things easier for the patients and those accompanying them as far as possible, and they even set up a kosher kitchen. But in spite of the foreseen difficulties, the missionaries underestimated the Jews' reaction. The Jewish community in Palestine used a variety of methods to draw back into its fold anyone who even appeared to be on the verge of converting to Christianity. Heavy social pressure was brought to bear on the candidate for conversion, going as far as to impose divorce, the removal of children from the parent's care, and finally excommunication. This meant the denial of the right to be buried in a Jewish cemetery and no part in the world to come. But above all, the community took advantage of the basis for its members' economic survival - charitable donations and their distribution - to deprive the convert of his source of subsistence.

Six weeks after the opening of the hospital, a patient died. The two Chief Rabbis in Jerusalem made his Jewish burial conditional on having all the patients in the hospital and all Jewish attendants leave immediately, and on a prohibition against any Jew entering the hospital's gates in the future. Several letters went back and forth for an entire week between the rabbis and the director of the hospital, and between the latter and the British Consul in Jerusalem and the Foreign Minister in London. The missionaries stood their ground and therefore were forced to bury the deceased patient in the British cemetery.[24] The seriousness of this event from the viewpoint of the Jerusalem rabbis induced them to take the gravest measure in their power without delay, and they issued a ban, worded as follows:

> All Israel shall hear and fear. As the horribleness in Israel upon Mount Zion, was clearly seen, from the affairs of the Freemasons' [sic] hospital, whose sole object wish & desire, by it, is to bring the souls of our brothers, of the house of Israel into their uncleanness … By the power of our holy law … we give notice that no man shall dare to enter the hospital above mentioned, whether a patient for his recovery, or a healthy person to serve there. Let both man & woman take warning by this our edict. We also inform all our brethren of the house of Israel that whosoever shall enter the said hospital; their meat & drink shall become, through a heavy excommunication as unlawful food -- their bread and wine shall become as the bread & wine of idolaters, all their children will not be circumcised (amongst the holy assembly, neither will he be called up to the reading of the law) nor shall

> he have any part in the God of Israel, he will also not be purified, after his decease, by Jews, nor buried in their burial ground. We caution also the Shokhatim [ritual slaughterers] of all the congregations, not to kill a fowl for those, of the house of Israel, who shall enter the hospital. Likewise we charge our vendors of meat, by the same powers, not to sell meat to any man or woman, who shall enter the hospital; should they, however, by any device, get meat from our vendors, then the dishes will be unlawful, the man or servant, through whom they got it, incurs the above mentioned curse. All the above mentioned curses shall be likewise upon every one, who will advise or induce any of the children of Israel, to enter the said hospital; but ye brethren, of the house of Israel, who cleave to the Lord, hear & your soul shall live. Whosoever shall transgress this our edict, renders himself liable to all the penalties above mentioned; but good blessings & prosperity will come upon those that hear our words. May the merits of our brethren of the house of Israel, & of Jerusalem our holy & glorious city defend us that none of us shall be led astray. Amen & so be the will of God![25]

Such a ban meant the excommunication of the person from the Jewish community or death by sheer deprivation. Within twenty-four hours of publication of this ban, the hospital was completely deserted. Yet in a few weeks the dismal medical conditions in Jerusalem appeared to dictate the position of the British Hospital in the town and the Jewish patients found their way back there. The hospital continued to function to the same standard for about fifty years. Every year hundreds of Jews were hospitalized and tens of thousands of visits to the dispensary were recorded.[26]

New Hospital in Jerusalem

In the mid-1870s, rumours began to spread in Jerusalem and London concerning the need for a new hospital because of the dilapidated state of the old hospital building and the increasing rate of occupancy. But only in September 1889 were the first decisions made regarding the site for the proposed building. The London Jews Society Committee in Jerusalem recommended that the hospital be built outside the city walls on a stretch of land acquired in 1863 on which the Society's recreation site, called the 'Sanatorium', would later be built. They envisaged the new institution as incorporating all the hospital facilities, including the dispensary and staff quarters, near the hospital wings. The old hospital building inside the city walls would be retained for use as outpatient clinics and a dispensary.

Beresford A. Pite (1861-1934), a British architect who was also a member of the London Jews Society, drafted the plans for the new hospital. The hospital was planned upon the pavilion or detached-ward principle, in which each ward is a self-contained and complete building, connected only to the general office of the hospital by covered corridors. The conditions of the location and the advantage of a full circulation of fresh air around and under each ward, as well as the possibility of completely isolating the wards, indicated the reasons for this arrangement. The hospital was to be divided into two sections – one for men and the other for women, with each section connected to the centre by the administrative offices. The outpatients' department would be located on one side of the entrance courtyard, and the nurses' premises and kitchens on the other side. Thus those sectors would be kept away from actual contact with the hospital itself. The flat roof, verandas and method of building adopted in Palestine were employed in the design.[27]

Pite arrived at his innovative design after much thought and following his extensive touring among similar institutions in Europe. He completed his assignment by the end of 1891 and, at the dedication ceremony of the building, Pite described the planning process:

> Three years ago funds were sufficient for an inspection to come out and survey the spot. I visited about twenty different hospitals at that time. The principles of the erection of the present hospital are simple, the main object being to cure patients with as little medicine as possible, and give them as much light and sunshine as we can. We all notice how many windows and doors the building contains.[28]

The new 'English Mission Hospital' for the Jews in Jerusalem, the flagship of the London Jews Society in Palestine and the institution

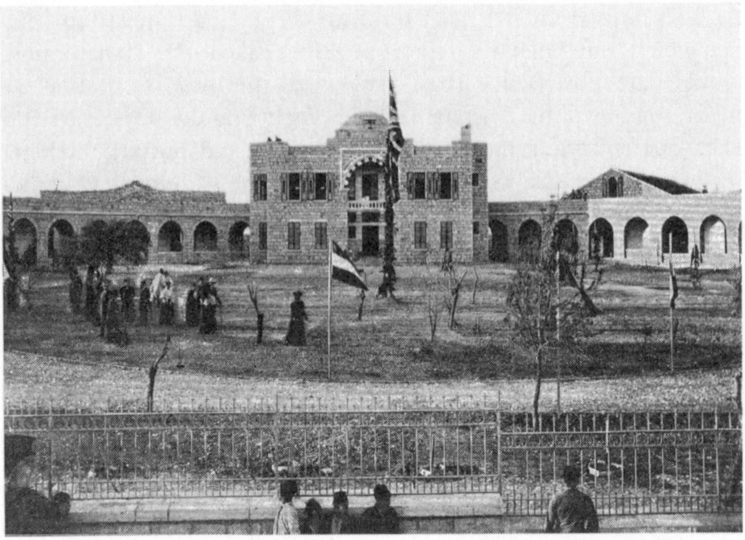

Figure 3 - Main building of the new hospital, Jerusalem, 1897

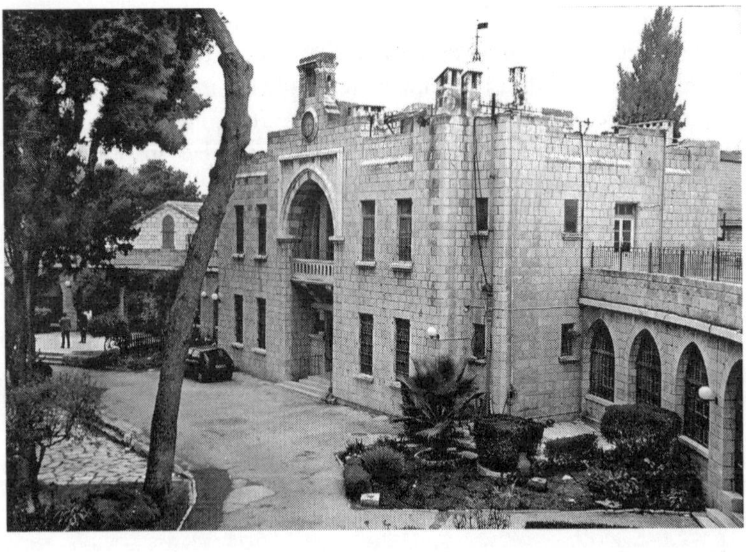

Figure 4 - Main building today (an Anglican School)

in which most of the funds and attention were invested, was inaugurated on April 13, 1897. Taking part in the festive ceremony were some of its leaders in England, Thomas Chaplin (1830-1904), who was the hospital director for twenty-five years, Consuls of foreign countries, heads of churches in Jerusalem, representatives of the Turkish government, all the London Jews Society members in Palestine. But not a single Jew was present.[29]

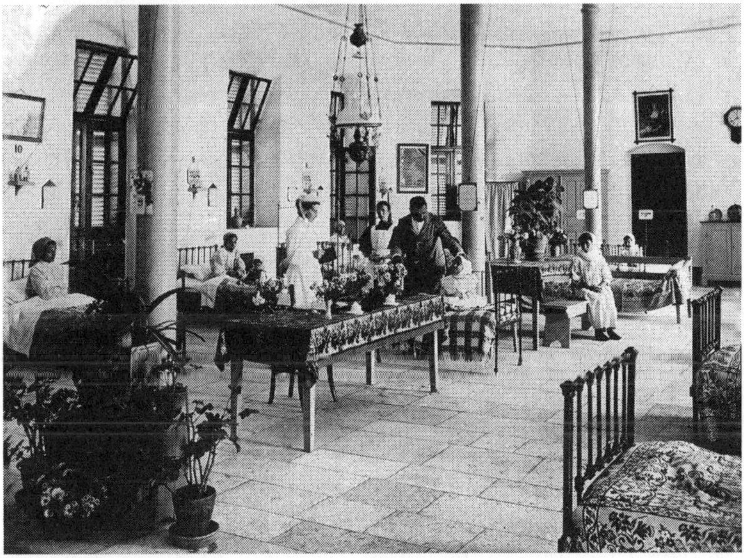

Figure 5 - Ward in the hospital, Jerusalem

For the reasons described above, the fact that not a single member of the Jewish community took part in the events held for the dedication of the hospital in Jerusalem was not a matter of chance. Its opening aroused fierce opposition, led mainly by an association called Bnei-Israel (Sons of Israel). It was founded in 1897 in reaction to the erection of the hospital. Influenced by the consensus of nearly all facets of the Jewish community, the association provided dispensaries and free medication for the welfare of the Jews in Jerusalem. Its avowed objective was to 'work for the unity of the congregations and for the improvement of the general situation'. However, in some cases, members of the Bnei-

Israel association were engaged in violent attempts to prevent the hospitalization of Jews in the English Mission Hospital for the Jews in Jerusalem.

It was not long before the Jewish sentries positioned at the gates of the hospital took violent physical measures, which caused the people in the medical establishment and the guards of the British Consulate to react. A few days later, in the wake of the riots both Her Majesty's Ambassador in Constantinople and the Foreign Office in London took up the entire matter. An appeal was made by Arthur Hastings Kelk (1835-1908), the head of the mission in Jerusalem, to the Jewish community in the Hebrew journal *Ha-Zevi*. The journal also published a summary of the clarifying talks held between Kelk and the community rabbis that contributed to a calming of spirits. Kelk said that he had no complaints against the rabbis, who were merely fulfilling their duty according to their faith, in dissuading the public from using the medical services of the Society; but he objected to the use of force.[30] Besides the violence employed against those visiting the hospital and sometimes against its employees, the members of Bnei-Israel used other means to eliminate the 'plague' called the British Hospital in Jerusalem. The fact that the institution was built outside the walls of the Old City, too far to maintain close supervision over those entering its gates, merely gave the members of the association added incentive for their actions. For example, the Bnei-Israel organization induced the Supreme Law Court of the Jewish community to publish in writing a sharp warning - one of many - that no Jew should use the services of the new hospital. The official declaration was as follows:

> We heads and leaders of the holy congregation... have unanimously decided to order a decree according to our rite, that it is unlawful for any shochet [ritual slaughterer] to kill either beast or fowl for the use of the aforenamed Hospital, likewise it is unlawful for any Israelite to sell, provide, or permit to be sold any Kosher meat to the aforesaid Hospital. This prohibition applies to the sellers who sell directly or indirectly, and whoever transgresses these our commands, if he be a shochet, whatever he killed will be considered 'Nebela' (beast that dieth of itself), and if he be a butcher, he will not

> be trusted to sell Kosher meat, and supply them [the hospital]. He will be dealt with according to our laws.[31]

Towards the end of the nineteenth century the London Jews Society added other buildings to the hospital to complete the original plan. In the spring of 1898 it instructed the hospital builder to continue with the construction of the Doctors' House at the site assigned for that purpose in the hospital's west wing. On July 11, 1901 the hospital was finished, together with the dedication of another wing named after the English philanthropist Richard Cadbury (1835-1899) of Birmingham, who had passed away in Jerusalem. So the construction of the grand medical institution, which later assumed a place of honour among the monumental nineteenth-century buildings in Jerusalem, was finally completed.

Hospital in Safed

Safed, being one of the four sacred cities of the Jewish people in Palestine and having a large Jewish population, was an obvious attraction for the London Jews Society. Attempts to settle in the city were made during exploratory expeditions of British missionaries in the 1820s, 1830s, and 1840s, but only following the first wave of Jewish immigration to Palestine during the 1880s did the Society renew its activities in full scale in this Galilean city. In the spring of 1884, a delegation set out from Jerusalem to facilitate matters for the opening of the Safed Mission Station and to post an emissary and a physician in the town.

Only in June 1893 did Dr Ernest Masterman (1867-1943), who served at the Jerusalem hospital and was transferred to Safed, send the London Jews Society leaders his impressions regarding the urgent need for a proper hospital:

> There is not one single Hospital in the whole town. Such a state of things does not exist elsewhere in Palestine. Practically, all the large towns in the country have well-appointed Medical Missions; but these are no good to those really ill in Safed, as a journey even to so near a place as the Scotch Mission [hospital] in Tiberias, can only be made by

> difficult mountain roads… Tiberias (4,000 inhabitants). Here the Scotch now have a Hospital, and are building a new and substantial one on the shores of the lake… In Nazareth (7,500 inhabitants), the Edinburgh Missionary Society has a long-established Medical Mission, with a small Hospital. At Nablous (20,000 inhabitants) [actually 13,000] the C.M.S. [Church Missionary Society] has a flourishing Medical Mission, only recently started, but with a Hospital and a salaried nurse. At Haifa (8,000 inhabitants), I understand our Bishop has a small Hospital attached to his Medical Mission. At Jaffa (23,000 inhabitants) there is, as you know, a long-established Medical Mission Hospital, with a large staff of nurses. The Roman Catholics also have a fine Hospital. At Hebron (10,000 inhabitants) Mrs. Meredith has also Hospital premises, and a Scotch doctor… is now at Constantinople taking his diploma preparatory to taking charge. The Jews are also building a small Hospital there. I quote the above to show that these towns (though all smaller than Safed) have well-appointed Medical Missions, with Hospitals; while we in Safed, though having so long established a work there have no Hospital, in spite of the fact of the needs being much greater.[32]

This strongly worded report reached London and attracted a great deal of attention. As a result of its publication, explicit instructions were issued directing that permission be obtained to build 'a small hospital' on land belonging to the London Jews Society in Safed. However, the success of the medical enterprise in the city led to a change of plan, and attempts were made to locate an additional plot of land to build a more spacious hospital. To carry out this project, Dr Walter Henry Anderson (1869-1937), a native of Burton-on-Trent in England, was appointed to head the medical department so that Masterman would be free to return to his duties in Jerusalem. As soon as Anderson arrived, in April 1894, he took up his post with great energy and declared that he saw his work in Safed as his life's vocation. His first recommendation was to open a small hospital of six beds immediately, and at the same time to continue with the efforts to build the projected large hospital. The

London Jews Society approved of his proposal, and at the end of 1895 he rented a building to be used as a hospital for a period of three years. It opened in February 1896.

In 1898, Anderson managed to obtain a license from the local authorities to build a residence for his family in the compound (bought in 1895) intended for a hospital with the hope of receiving, in time, permission for building the hospital itself. He also reported to the London Jews Society that at the end of June he had signed an agreement with Gottlieb Schumacher (1857-1925), a German building consultant in Haifa, for constructing the residence. Schumacher was asked to start planning the hospital as well, and towards the end of 1899 he completed the first draft of his plans for the new medical institution and sent them for review to the Society leaders. At the end of May 1903 the construction work commenced.

At first, progress was very slow, and Anderson sent a letter from Safed complaining of the distress suffered at the temporary hospital. He emphasized the urgent need for speeding up the building of the permanent medical institution:

> I only wish I had the power vividly to bring before the Committee the misery of continuing to carry on the work in the present most wretched premises... At the present time I am obliged to perform surgical operations in the wards with a screen round the operation table! The so-called operation room defies description; the walls are reeking with damp, and the plaster falling off in all directions... If the new Hospital is not ready for occupation by the time winter has well commenced, I shall have to definitely advise the Committee to close that branch of the Medical work temporarily.[33]

A few months later, Anderson once more complained about the state of the temporary hospital and noted that the rental agreement for the building was to expire in September. He claimed that because of its dilapidated condition, the building would no longer serve his purpose even if the lease were extended for another year. Therefore, he recommended renting another temporary building until the expected opening of the new medical institution in the summer of 1904, or alternatively, to close down the medical ward

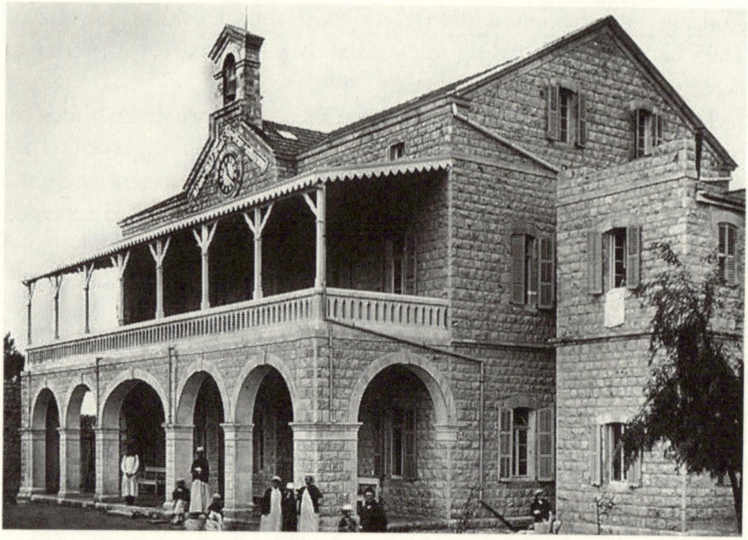

Figure 6 - Hospital in Safed 1912?

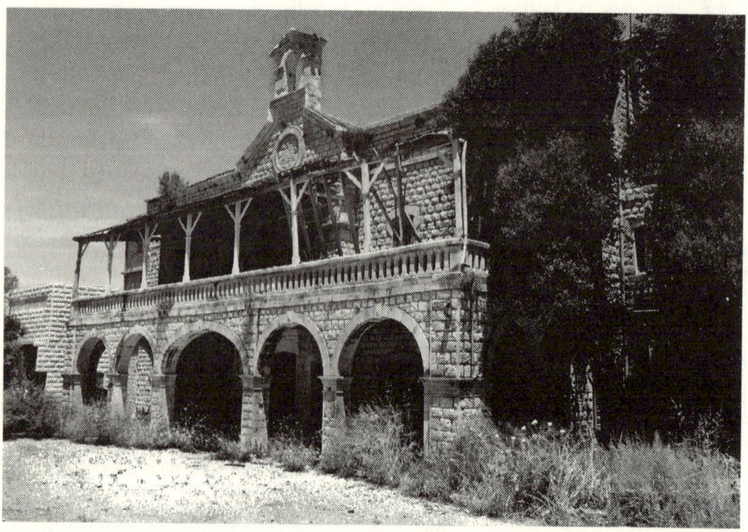

Figure 7 - Hospital in Safed today

completely.[34] From another letter Anderson sent to London, it appears that in the autumn of 1903 his April foreboding had come to pass. The doctor preferred not to continue using the damp and decrepit building any longer, since, in his words, it was better, in the winter season, to place the patients outside the institution, under the open sky. Medical activity ceased and efforts were made to find another temporary building for rent while the permanent building was being completed.

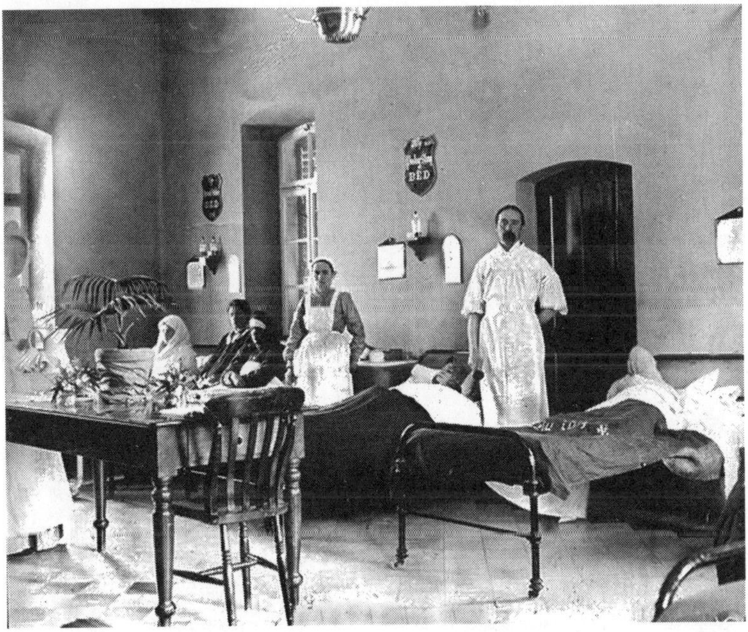

Figure 8 - Female ward in Safed, 1906

On May 31, 1904, the new hospital was inaugurated in Safed. The four-storey building was equipped with the best medical equipment available and contained hospital wards for forty men and women, a modern operating theatre and a kosher kitchen. This modern institution fired the imagination of the editor of the Society's journal in London. He published an article penned by Anderson, describing in great detail every aspect of the institution, taking the readers on a complete tour of the interior:

> Upon entering we are at once struck by its brightness and English-like appearance. The floors are composed of white cement tiles, with a border of black. The walls are tinted a soft, pink colour. The modern English fireplace, with turquoise blue tiles and white enamelled mantel-piece, at once arrests the attention of the English traveller, who has probably not seen the like since leaving the homeland.[35]

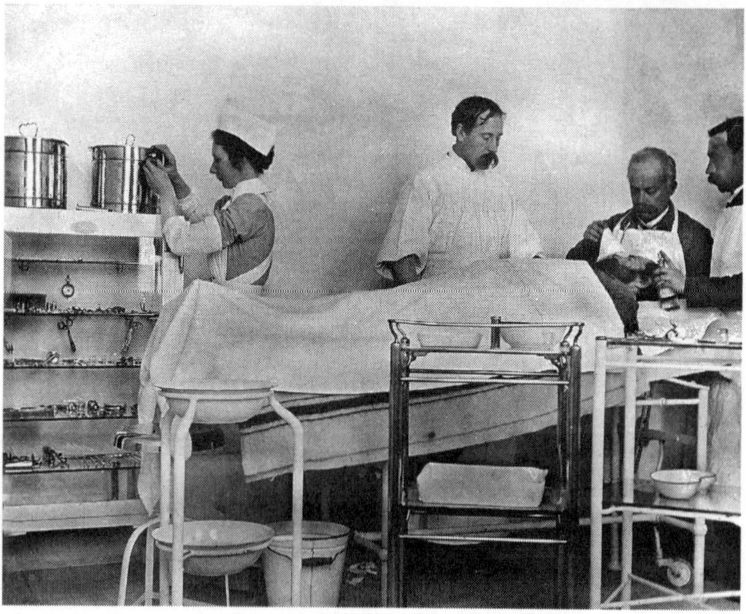

Figure 9 - Anderson in the operating room

At the dedication ceremony, for the very first time at an event of this kind, many of the Jews of Safed participated since the hospital was the only medical institution in the city, which also served the Jews in the Galilee settlements. A few years later Anderson, in a speech in London on the situation at his medical institute, gave a clear analysis of the attitude of the Jewish community towards the hospital. He summed it up in a single sentence: 'A few years ago the difficulty with us was how to get at these fanatical people in Safed; now the difficulty is not how to get at them, but how to get away from them'.[36] Obviously, he was exaggerating, but the spirit of good will towards the Jews, which allowed them continuous use of the hospital, prevailed in Safed.

The extent of the hospital's success can be gathered from a Jewish ban publicly displayed in Safed:

> In our city the work of the mission is more than in any of the holy cities; the enticers labour day and night, and use every means to draw our brethren to them, especially the young. Their doctors heal all Jewish patients gratis, as if the Christian religion enjoins to pity only [emphasis in original] the Jewish poor, and by this means about fifty Jews (even of the most pious) listen daily to the addresses from the preachers, causing them to go astray...[37]

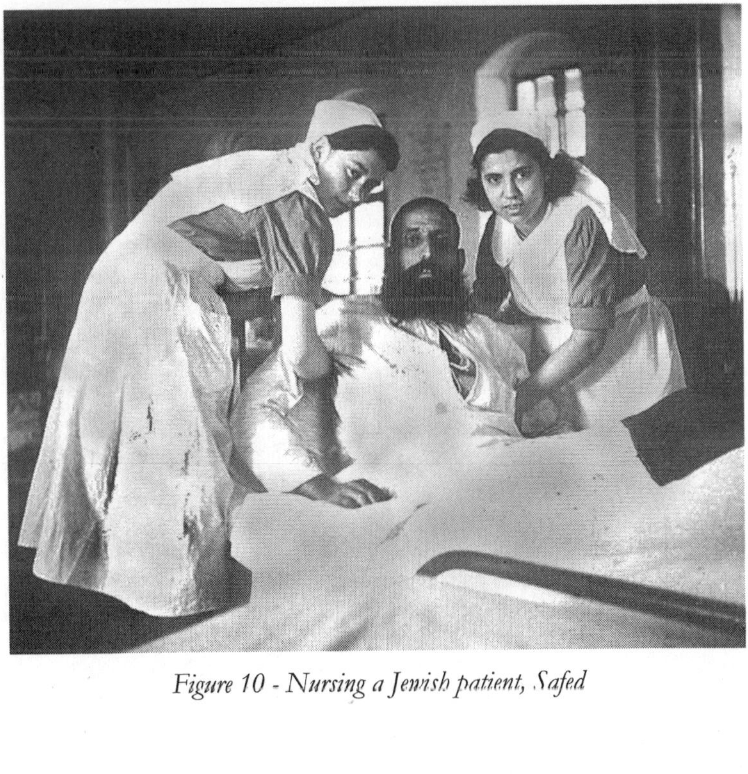

Figure 10 - Nursing a Jewish patient, Safed

Pharmacological and Medical Aspects

Britain, as a colonial power, provided advanced medical services for its citizens who were stationed as government officials, military personnel, or merchant traders in every corner of the globe. As proof of this, the medical press in England ran regular columns with reports on British medical activities around the world, a 'wanted' column for engaging doctors and pharmacists for medical work in the colonies, and even accounts of military medicine around the world. Detailed and accurate reports were part of the culture of governing which made the existence of a colonial empire possible. This had been an ingrained feature of British colonial practice for centuries, and the medical missionaries serving in the Jerusalem hospitals acted in keeping with it. Although the hospital functioned as a private institution belonging to a philanthropic organization, strict regulations on keeping of records and drawing up reports were observed.

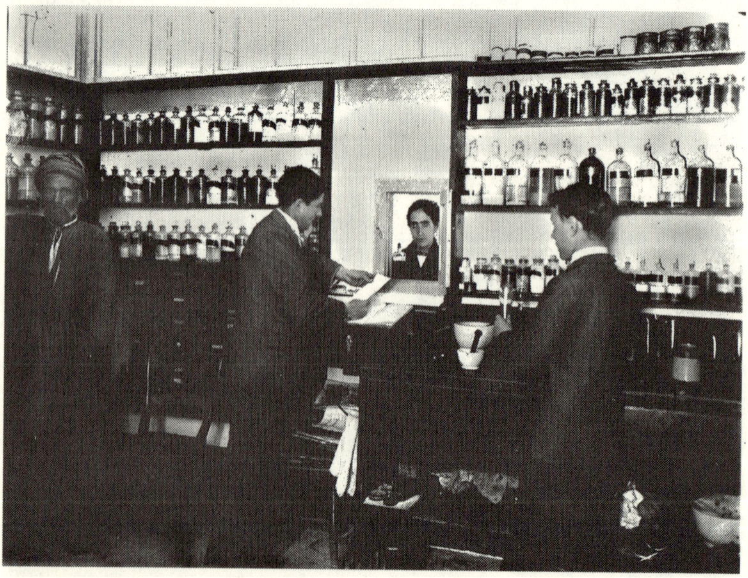

Figure 11 - Dispensers at work, Jerusalem

The medical activities of the London Jews Society in Jerusalem are recorded in its rich archives deposited in the Bodleian Library at Oxford. There many documents relating to medical activities in the society's hospitals in Palestine were drawn upon, including medical reports, plans for the construction of medical institutions, personnel matters and publications concerning these institutions, as well as extensive correspondence for data related to this research. This chapter presents one document out of the London Jews Society archival collection that throws light upon the medical methods practised in the early period of the hospital. It is an inventory of medications in the store of the dispensary at the Jerusalem hospital, dated 1857. It lists 266 items on nine pages in partially legible handwriting and is entitled 'List of Medicinal Preparations Found in Store and Dispensary on July 21, 1857'.[38] Table 1 summarises its composition.

Table 1. Medicinal Substances in the British Hospital, Jerusalem 1857

Type of Product	Number
Oils	29
Liquid preparations	9
Acids	16
Alkalis and salts	23
Metallic salts	46
Alkaloidal salts	13
Gums	11
Extracts	23
Pills	2
Ointments	8
Powders	42
Roots, barks, leaves	31
Aethers [sic.] and spirits	13
Total	**266**

Data Analysis

Special attention should be paid, over and above all the other materials, to the ether and chloroform, both found in the last group of materials in Table 1 (aethers [sic.] and Spirits). Their presence might be strong evidence of the first application of modern techniques of anaesthesia in the Holy Land. Until 1999 it might have been considered evidence of the first surgical use of chloroform in the Ottoman Empire, since previously the first known use was in 1864, but new chronological research into the annual reports of the Galatasaray Medical School in Istanbul, revealed that the first surgical use of chloroform in the Ottoman Empire was actually at the Imperial Medicine School at Galatasaray in 1848.[39]

Analysis reveals the sources of the drugs and preparations:

Table 2. Composition of the 1857 list of medicinal preparations

Source	No. of substances	Percentage
Plants	157	59.0
Chemicals and minerals	104	39.1
Animals	5	1.9
Total	**266**	**100**

Comparisons with other lists

A comparative examination showed that the list contains a quarter of the *materia medica* known and applied in that period in England,[40] and altogether about a third of the items in the *British Pharmacopoeia* of 1858, which contained 734 medicines.[41] Similarly, a comparison of the list with the standard inventory of clinics in nineteenth century England shows that the stores of the hospital and clinic in Jerusalem contained about 80% of the substances used at that time.[42] Most of the raw materials for preparing the medicines were imported from England, including those found in abundance in Palestine, both in the open fields and in the city markets. Among the substances derived from plants were several originating in Asia, mainly in India (Cajuput), Africa (Kino), and the Americas (Cinchona, Ipecacuanha, Sassafras). The use of substances from the New World was a characteristic of modern medicine, and the only evidence of such substances present in the Levant at the time is of quinine, used by the Franciscan monks in Jerusalem as early as the eighteenth century.[43] The only animal substances located in this list are cod liver oil, cetaceum (spermaceti), sperm oil, Spanish fly (cantharides - for blistering and as an aphrodisiac), lard and animal charcoal. These substances were widely used in the past as medications and are prevalent today in traditional medicine practised throughout the Middle East. For comparison, note that in that region during the Middle Ages the use of substances from 30 different kinds of animals has been recorded in the framework of scholarly medicine.[44]

Many of the substances found in the list could have been obtained in the Jerusalem marketplace. For example, cinnamon, nutmeg, pepper, camphor, aloe vera, sulphur, gall-nut, lead, iron, zinc, gum-arabic, galbanum, pine resin, soap, myrrh, rhubarb, cardamom and galanga. Also listed were substances that could be found plentifully both in nature and in Palestinian agriculture, such as castor oil, almond, water melon, bitter apple, bindweed, liquorice, pistachio, squill and laburnum.

Additional plants appearing in the list could easily have been grown in the garden of the English Mission Hospital in Jerusalem: rosemary, lavender, basil, anise, and saffron. The founder of the hospital, Dr Edward Macgowan, made a proposal on this matter in February 1842. In his efforts to establish the hospital, he urged the London Jews Society leaders to allow him to lease a plot of land and to employ a local worker to cultivate a garden adjoining the institution. Thus, 'it would be possible for the Medical Department to save expenses by growing medicinal plants.[45] However, even if the hospital staff were to raise these plants in their garden, or collect them from the open fields, there would still be the need to extract the oils, to produce the powders, to collect the resinous juices and so on. Such processes need professional skills, expensive training and reliable workers over a prolonged period of time. The medical staff undoubtedly preferred to purchase the oils, essences and powders in England, where these substances were produced in mass quantities by industrial processes and were of the highest quality of the time.

The reasons against purchasing these products in England might be the distance between Jerusalem hospital and London, the methods of transport, and the risk thus incurred to the medicinal substances and medications. A consignment took several weeks to arrive by ship from England, and after arrival it was transported from the port of Jaffa to Jerusalem by mule caravans. Another possible explanation could have been the financial situation of the London Jews Society, which enabled it to purchase only the primary basic substances. The traditional substances in the medical stores of the English Mission Hospital in Jerusalem, constituting more than half of the listed items, were apparently a significant factor in the inventory of substances, so their medical importance was therefore relatively high. These substances seem gradually to have disappeared, and are hardly mentioned in the pharmacological framework of conventional medicine. However, they did not disappear entirely and some were to occupy a major place in the stores of alternative medicine, which is very popular today among the sick and ailing.

A comparison of the inventory listing with the list of popular medicinal substances drawn up, as described above, by Tobler after his visit to Jerusalem in 1845, also proves that the substances in the Jerusalem markets and in the city dispensaries, such as the Jewish, Greek and Franciscan dispensaries, could have been of help to the British Hospital in time of need (Table 3). Among the 57 substances of plant origin we find herbs such as rosemary and chamomile, and spices such as cinnamon, ginger and clove. The list also contains resins and gums such as tragacanth, sarcocolla and myrrh, roots such as spikenard, rhubarb, sweet-violet, seeds and fruits such as myrobalan and bitter-vetch and different oils: black pepper oil, caraway oil, nutmeg oil and many others.

As for minerals, Tobler describes nine in his list, most of which were different kinds of salts such as borax, English salt and tartar; pure minerals such as sulphur and other substances of mineral origin such as the 'armenische Bolus' (Armenian bole).[46] Of the eight substances of animal origin described by Tobler, two were derived from the beaver: *Bibergeil* (beaver gland) and the Arabic term *Dehen el-Mannasar* (oil of beaver gland).[47] Tobler added that 'One of the most unique substances was the 'Mumie' (local name); the inhabitants believed it has an exceptional curing power'.[48] This substance was the remains of bodies, mainly of Egyptian mummies, which was sold in the markets of Jerusalem. The mummies were used by members of all faiths to cure people who were dying, and as of 2007 the material may still be purchased at one shop in the Old City of Jerusalem.[49]

Tobler added that he heard about the oil of the 'Zaqum', which according to him cured 'wounds within days'. 'A Venetian traveller who fell off his horse felt a worrying ache in his chest, rubbed his body with 'Zaqum' oil and drank some, and within some days the wound was scarred over and the internal aches were eased'.[50] *Zaqum* is the Arabic and Hebrew name for Egyptian balsam (*Balanites aegyptiaca*), a tropical tree that grows wild in the Judean desert, in the Eastern part of Israel. The oil pressed out of its fruit has been used as a medicine since early history.[51] Tobler also mentioned the frequent use of Theriac,[52] which is a mixture of many medicinal substances: plants, poisonous minerals and extracts of generally poisonous animals, such as snakes and scorpions.[53] The manufacturing process for Theriac was a well-kept secret throughout history. Medieval Muslim medicine made use of a different kind of Theriac such as the Jerusalem Theriac which was famous for its medicinal qualities and was even exported to other countries.[54]

Table 3. Composition of Tobler's List of Medicinal Materials

Origin/Source	No. of substances	Percentage
Plants	57	70.4
Minerals	9	11.1
Animals	8	9.9
Other	7	8.6
Total	**81**	**100**

Comparison of the total number of drugs in the 1857 list (table 2) with the total number of drugs of the inventory of medicinal substances in the al-Sham region (i.e., the Levant: Israel and parts of Syria, Lebanon and Jordan today) during the medieval and early Ottoman period was made and found to be similar (Table 4). Comparison between the 1857 listing and the historical inventory of medicinal substances in the lengthy time-span from the Muslim conquest in the seventh century to Napoleon's campaign at the end of the eighteenth century shows a decline in the number of plants used as a basis for medications from 234 to 157 (plants were often used as sources of chemical compounds) and in the number of animal-based products from 30 to 5. In the 1857 listing, 104 chemicals and minerals were used — a new and significant factor in the inventory of medicines. These in fact replaced the minerals used in the medicines of earlier periods until the Middle Ages and generally constituted 5-10% of the general inventory. This comparison of the historical inventory and conventional listings is introduced here for the sole purpose of assessment.

Table 4. Medicinal Substances used in the Levant during the Medieval and Early Ottoman Period

Origin	Number	Percentage
Plants	234	81.8
Animals	27	9.5
Minerals	15	5.2
Others	10	3.5
Total	**286**	**100**

The overwhelming majority of substances that served as simple drugs or as a basis for complex drugs derived from plants. The proportion of materials derived from animals and animal organs was small. Minerals represented only a small proportion of the medieval list, either because of their relatively small number in nature, or because great caution was exercised in the application of minerals and chemical substances uncommon in daily use. Considered from a comparative perspective, these statistics resemble the distribution of substances found in lists of medicinal substances from different periods and cultures.[55]

A botanical analysis revealed plant species whose medicinal use in the region was previously uncertain or unknown. These plants include: common agrimony (*Agrimonia eupatoria*), deer balls (*Lycoperdon* sp.), Christmas rose (*Helleborus* sp.), common gromwell (*Lithospermum officinale*), gardenia (*Gardenia* sp.), Job's tears (*Coix lachryma-jobi*), Solomon's seal (*Polygonatum officinale*), common yew (*Taxus baccata*), dodder (*Cuscuta* sp.), great snapdragon (*Antirrhinum malus*), squirting cucumber (*Momordica balsamina*), small caltrops (*Tribulus terrestris*), great horsetail (*Equisetum telmateia*) and the drias plant (*Thapasia gargenica*).

Several plants traced in the historical sources were used in keeping with an ancient medical theory — called in the late Middle Ages the 'Doctrine of Signatures', (a theory that asserts that the way plants, animals and minerals look, feel, taste or react suggests their medicinal application). Plants such as: lemon balm (*Melissa officinalis*), coral peony (*Paeonia* sp.), tanning sumach (*Rhus coriaria*), corn gromwell (*Lithospermum officinale*), great snapdragon, horned poppy (*Glaucium corniculatum*), spiny broom (*Calicotome villosa*), southern maidenhair fern (*Adiantum capillus-veneris*) and wild dog rose (*Rosa canina*) were used to treat symptoms and diseases which were similar in colour, shape or effects.[56] The animals traced in the historical sources can be divided into groups according to their availability:

1. Domesticated animals such as cattle *(Bos taurus)* and chickens (*Gallus galus domesticus*), pests such as lice (*Pediculus* sp.) and stinking bug (*Cimex lectularius*), and others such as the earthworm (*Lumbricus* sp.) and the firefly (*Lampyris* sp.). The use of these animals, their organs, and products is explained by their immediate availability, which made possible fresh supplies at low cost.
2. Wild animals such as the poisonous snake adder (*Echis coloratus*), the amphibious triton (*Titurus vittatus*) and the common beaver (*Castor fiber*).
3. Exotic animal species such as musk (*Moschus moschiferus*) and coral (*Coralium rubrum*).[57]

Seventeen substances of mineral origin have been traced in the medieval and early Ottoman historical sources. One of the conclusions drawn is that most of these medicinal substances were mined and produced in the Levant. The majority of such substances were geologically related to the Red Sea Rift in the southern part of Israel, while the remainder was found primarily in the northern part of the country.[58]

It is instructive to compare the medical services of the London Jews Society in nineteenth century Palestine, with the level of medical services provided by the Ottoman medical system decades earlier, and even with the services provided by the Franciscan medical institution. The comparison shows that the British started a new era in Palestine, that of modern medicine. One of the best pieces of historical evidence of the turning point in the medical history of Palestine is a list compiled in July 1857 of medicinal substances stored in the hospital dispensary in Jerusalem. The document is one of the first written testimonies of modern medical and pharmacological activity in the Levant in general and Palestine in particular. For millennia the lists of medicinal substances which were used by humans contained a fixed proportion of substances according to their origin (plants, minerals and animals). The composition of the 1857 list testifies above all to the increasing use of various chemicals as medicines or as components together with plants, minerals and animal substances. The growing use of chemicals and minerals was at the expense of substances derived from animals and of other indefinite origins, which had been more prevalent in the past. The presence of chloroform and ether in the list might be strong evidence for the first application in the Holy land of modern techniques of anaesthesia.

THE BRITISH PHYSICIANS

The English doctors were the first modern European physicians who practiced medicine in nineteenth century Palestine in general and Jerusalem in particular. They managed to function under very difficult conditions, far away from their homeland and equally distant from their accustomed civilization and modernity. They endangered their lives and sometime even lost their wives and children. They faced harsh physical conditions and a demanding practice e.g. treating up to a hundred patients during the day and writing detailed reports to the London Jews Society back home at night. All of them worked in a tense political, international, inter religion and inter ethnic milieu. In order to practice in Palestine, the English physicians had to be either very religious and devoted to their missionary work, or motivated by their curiosity and adventurousness (or both). Another obstacle in the way of the physicians was the patients' lack of understanding of healthy life style habits and of good medical practices. This unfortunately, was true of all types of patients; Jews, Muslims and local Christians. The need for medical help among the local inhabitants of the Holy Land was enormous. Superstitions against surgery, vaccination and injections were particularly prevalent.[1] Therefore, the London Jews Society sought physicians 'whose piety and other qualifications are suitable', those 'other qualifications' included demonstrating kindness and a pleasant personality.[2] Most physicians, beginning with Edward Mcgowan, dealt with fundraising and had the ability to elicit charitable donations as well. They collected clothing in England for distribution among the poor Jews that visited the dispensary. In days to come a formal 'Hospital Relief Fund' was established to collect funds and clothing for the patients.[3]

The missionary physicians in Palestine functioned together with the authority of the head of the mission station. These roles – missionary and physician – had competing demands, and regulations became necessary to resolve the conflicts. James Elder Cumming, a Scottish clergyman and scholar, took this matter under consideration in his writings more than once. In a Scottish missionary paper he wrote that the work of the medical missionary is not a mission, but a branch of a mission. He must have beside him a clergyman, whose duty is to preach, and who often must 'enter in where the physician has opened the way'.[4]

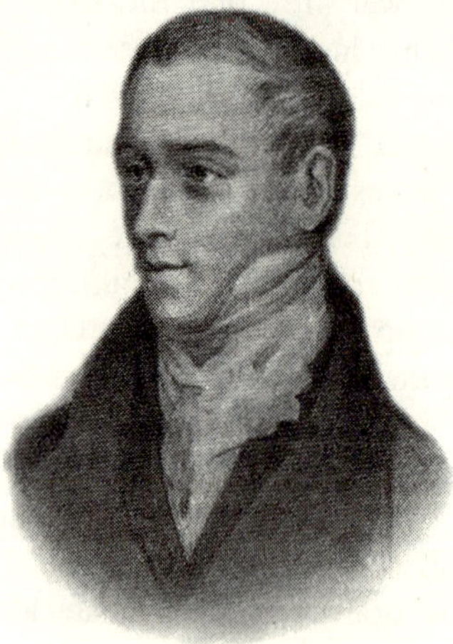

Figure 12 - Dr George Edward Dalton

Sometimes, when several missionaries operated in one mission station, the physician overshadowed his colleagues. In most cases in Palestine, besides acting as head of the medical institution, the physician became well known as a scholar as well. The physicians also had to have, in Cummings words, some practical knowledge of the 'apothecary's business; much more than are needed in an ordinary practice at home'. In these circumstances, the heads of the London Jews Society sometimes worried that the roles of physician and medical scholar would replace the role as missionary. At all times, the role as a missionary was supposed to be of greater importance than any other. Thus, the missionary physician could contribute to international medical journals, but first and foremost he must be a

> 'Christian man, with the love of Christ in his heart, with some power to teach, and with some love for teaching – not merely ready to use opportunities that may occur, but anxious to find or to make them – not to preach publicly, but to explain and to teach, and to press home the Gospel message to sinful men'.[5]

Dr Edward Macgowan (1795-1860)

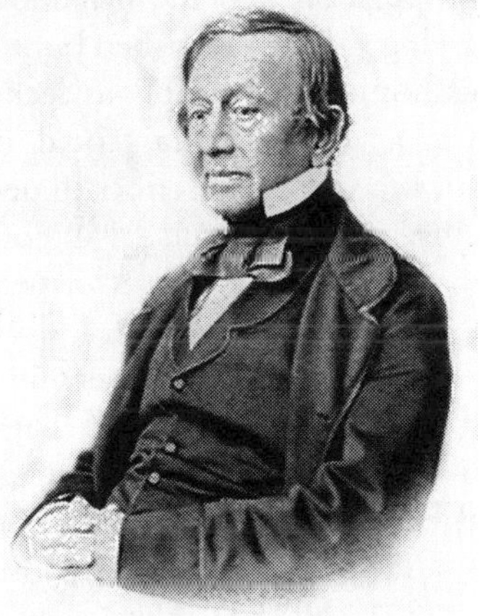

Figure 13 - Dr Edward Macgowan

Dr Edward Macgowan was born in 1795. In 1841, when he was 46 and a well-established physician in Exeter, he joined the London Jews Society with the aim of founding the first modern hospital in Palestine. The first attempt by the Society to establish a medical missionary in Palestine in the 1820s failed because the first physician they sent, Dr George Edward Dalton, died. Early in 1841, the Society's principals resolved to execute plans for founding a hospital for the Jews. They published in their journal a notice, encouraging readers to communicate with the committee if they were acquainted with a 'gentleman whose piety and other qualifications are suitable'.[6] It seems that Dr Edward Macgowan was recommended to the committee soon thereafter. The committee concluded that 'His professional character stands too high to make it necessary for him to transmit his Testimonials'.[7] On December 7, 1841 Macgowan sailed from Portsmouth aboard the *Devastation.* On the voyage to Palestine the vessel called in at Lisbon, Gibraltar, Malta and Beirut. On January 21, 1842 Macgowan arrived in the city of Jerusalem.[8]

Professional work as a physician

Macgowan began work immediately upon arrival in Jerusalem. While making arrangements for a place of residence, he acquainted himself with the population and the neighbourhood. He devoted each morning to seeing the impoverished poor in their homes or by appointment at his home. Within only a week of arrival he had as many applications for advice as he could manage. In his first account to London, Macgowan describes in detail the poor state of health of the Jerusalem Jews and also complained about the building that was rented to serve as a dispensary and about the shortage of surgical instruments and drugs. Macgowan urged the committee to press for the establishment of a hospital and for additional medical assistance.[9] He implied that it would be possible to economise on the expenses of the medical department by growing medicinal herbs, and exhorted the society to let him rent some land for this purpose and to employ a local worker.[10]

In the first six months of 1842, Macgowan established his work with the Jerusalem population on a regular basis. Even the resultant opposition from the city's Jewish establishment was low-key, and Macgowan himself wrote to London that he wondered at the absurdity of reports of the opposition and insults that he was said to have endured. He stated that since his arrival in Jerusalem, he had not experienced any annoyance or disrespect from either the public authorities or the inhabitants. Moreover, in the spring he received many requests for medical advice from the local Muslim physicians as well:[11] 'We are going on wonderfully well in Jerusalem', he wrote.[12] Along with this optimism Macgowan gives details of the diseases peculiar to the country - eye diseases, cataract, intermittent fevers, ague (due to the lack of cleanliness of the reservoir), visceral obstructions, dropsies (chronic), typhus, diarrhoea and dysentery.[13]

In the following year Macgowan encountered, in his own words, 'much inconvenience and suffering'. Because of the disorder that prevailed in the country, in July 1843 he was attacked by Turkish soldiers. On his way to Bethlehem, passing through the bazaar, some soldiers began to beat his horse. In trying to fend off the assault he was beaten himself:

> I was in the midst of a dense crowd, from which it was impossible to extricate myself ... Among them I noticed several Jews who were struggling with the soldiers and striving to get me out of their hands. I shall never forget the courageous assistance they afforded me on that occasion, to which, in all probability, my preservation, humanly speaking, is owing.[14]

The maltreatment affected Macgowan for most of the year. He was ailing during the autumn and spent much time in Hebron and Bethlehem for change of scenery. In January 1844, he was back on duty and working as usual.[15]

Founding the hospital

On December 12, 1844 the English Mission Hospital was opened to serve the sick, destitute and despised Jews in Jerusalem.[16] The missionary orientation of the hospital was well known to the leaders of the Jewish community in Jerusalem and it raised heavy opposition. Macgowan tried to make things as easy as possible for the patients, even setting up a kosher kitchen, but he still had to face the Jewish antagonism. Nonetheless, patients came to the hospital, slowly at first and then more. Early in 1848 Macgowan described the progress of the mission's medical department by pointing out that some respectable Jews of a higher class presented themselves in his waiting-room. In his opinion this showed how fully the original prejudice against the hospital had worn away, replaced by confidence in the ability and good intentions of the Jews' benefactors.[17] Two years later Macgowan shared his impressions in the Society's journal: the hospital had never stood its ground so well. 'It is even patronized by some of the most influential Jews ... I never expected to meet with the gratitude which is shown by the poor Jews, and am delighted with their excellent behaviour when inmates'.[18]

A year later Macgowan was proud to report the visit by the Chief Rabbi of Jerusalem who fell ill with fever and was admitted to the hospital. During that visit Macgowan observed that the Rabbi's daughter had a squint in her right eye. Macgowan operated on the girl successfully and reported this as the first operation of its kind to be performed in Jerusalem.[19] Operations on patients in those early days in Jerusalem were not a daily occurrence. The meagre skills of the local physicians increased the Eastern prejudice against surgery. From time to time Macgowan's assistant had to undo the work of those procedures himself and he found the 'remedy was far worse than the disease'.[20] A few months later a report in the Society's journal stated that indeed great prejudice hereto had existed in the East on the subject of surgery. Yet owing to the confidence many felt in Macgowan, these notions were very often overcome and consequently many lives were saved.[21]

Superstition within the Jewish community was another matter Macgowan had to overcome during his tenure as head of the mission's medical institute in Jerusalem. He observed the prevalence of popular belief in magic and witchcraft in cases of epilepsy, melancholy, convulsions and aberration of mind. The Jews frequently turned to Muslim sorcerers, convinced that those affected were possessed by evil spirits. The spirits, it was thought, could be cast out by certain charms, amulets and incantations, which those 'impostors' pretend to know. Macgowan reported a visit he made to the Jewish hospital at a time when a revered Rabbi's wife was a patient there. The woman's family had compelled the Jewish physician to have a Muslim sorcerer present. Macgowan was allowed to come and he watched the magic treatment for casting out on evil spirit in that hospital. He gives a detailed account of the event, including insight into the establishment and its patients. He concludes: 'I am in hopes that least useful result of this case will be, to open the eye of the family and persons interested, and to shake their belief in the efficacy of charms and sortileges'.[22]

Five years later Macgowan informed readers of the Society's journal of another kind of superstitious notion in the practice of medicine in Palestine. One time he allowed a patient's wife to visit him at the hospital once a day instead of once a week which was the general rule. She availed herself of the opportunity to give her husband a dose of mummy, a remedy believed to possess extraordinary powers.

Relations with the Jewish community

Macgowan managed to establish a close relationship with Jerusalem's Jewish community and some of its leaders. The treatment he offered the suffering Jews combined with his friendly personality, made that relationship possible. Because of his daily contacts with Jews from all classes, Macgowan knew a great deal about their inner feelings, distress and conflicts. Several times he describes the distress owing to years of drought and scarcity of provisions. In his accounts, Macgowan writes of the families of respected Rabbis who were not ashamed of applying for relief. Macgowan reported, that in the 1840s, for the first time, some of the poorest took to begging in the streets, rather than relying on the Jewish welfare system. Macgowan concludes his report by telling readers about the additional role of the hospital, in providing for the substantial needs of the Jews as well. In a vivid description of his new medical institution, he writes about distinguishing patients who really require medical advice from those who suffer from want. The most needy approached the hospital's matron who gave from her stores articles of clothing, flour and a little money, according to the wants of the applicant.[23] Sometimes Macgowan himself took money from his private resources, which included donations from friends in England for distribution as he determined appropriate, to purchase flour for his most destitute patients.[24]

Macgowan maintained friendly relations with his Jewish professional colleagues. When his hospital was about to be opened in Jerusalem, the British Jew Moses Montefiore financed the construction of a Jewish hospital in Jerusalem. In addition, in mid-1843 Dr Shimon Fränkel arrived in Jerusalem to assist in the operation of the hospital.[25] Shortly after, the two physicians met and Macgowan reported that he considered the Jewish doctor a real advantage in providing medical relief to the poor Jews in Jerusalem.[26] Two months later Macgowan wrote to London that Fränkel had established a dispensary and begun to practise among the Jews:

> I see him frequently and have found him a kindly disposed and well-informed man. His practice however, has not relieved me of any portion of my own labours among the Jews; for the number of my patients has rather increased than fallen off...[27]

In his relations with the Jews of Jerusalem, Macgowan fulfilled his missionary function as well. He regularly visited synagogues of all Jewish congregations and was able to use his acquaintance with different communities for missionary purposes. He described the North African Jews (Mograbi), whose share in the general distribution of provisions in the Jewish community was neglected, and he recognized their wish to constitute themselves as a separate and independent body. He observed they were independent of the Rabbinical authorities, much more than any other group in Palestine. Moreover, unlike the other Jews, the North Africans were mostly French subjects and not under Turkish jurisdiction. Converting them to Christianity would not incur the same civil and ecclesiastical difficulties as in converting other Jews. He wrote 'They are poor, ignorant, despised, and neglected by all the world. What a blessing would infant schools and Christian instruction be to these poor outcast of the seed of Abraham'.[28]

A pioneer in researching the Holy Land

Macgowan was the first British physician in the English Mission Hospital to conduct research of the Holy Land. He showed keen research skills from his first year in Palestine. He gave accounts of the main diseases and sanitary conditions in the country, found the energy to tour and survey the country, and sent regular reports regarding the conditions in the Arab villages and described their treatment of Muslim patients. In one of his visits to the north of the Holy Land he analysed its geological nature and the character and habits of the Jews. Macgowan found time to perform climate monitoring as well. He made a daily record of barometric measurements, including temperatures and winds. He attached some of these records to his detailed reports to London and some were published in the Society's journal.[29]

Dr Edward Macgowan was the most important of the early British physicians in Jerusalem from the 1830s. Being in the van of a series of physicians, he built the dispensary and the hospital in the city, established connections with the local Ottoman regime, contended with Rabbinical bans and won the trust of the members of the Jewish community.

The physicians and surgeons who performed under Macgowan as director of the medical mission until 1860 were devoted employees and with little spare time for other activities. Some reported to the mission committee in London and their reports were frequently published in the Society's journal, but did nothing more. Macgowan's successor, Dr Thomas Chaplin, worked in a different atmosphere, generated and nurtured by Macgowan: by the time Chaplin assumed his post in Jerusalem, the hospital was established; the medical staff was organized and functioned smoothly; the health of the mission members was better; the local Ottoman authorities supported the hospital's work; and the dispute with the Jerusalem Rabbis was moderated.[30]

Edward Macgowan died in Jerusalem on Monday, February 6, 1860 and was buried in the Protestant cemetery on Mount Zion. His friends and colleagues in Jerusalem described the suffering he faced during his illness, and the manner in which he bore it with exemplary patience and resignation.[31] He become very spiritual in his last few months and he, a highly educated man with a large library, cared nothing for his books during his last illness. He could speak very little. Nothing seemed to comfort him but a 'simple text of Scripture' brightened him up and he would often complete it himself. Macgowan achieved a significant undertaking in Jerusalem. Thousands of Jews in Palestine bore witness to this when they cried out 'A prince and a great man is fallen in Israel'.[32]

Dr Thomas J. Chaplin (1830-1904)

For a quarter of a century, Dr Thomas J. Chaplin was the director of the British hospital for the Jews in Jerusalem, in the service of the London Jews Society. He improved the medical situation in the city, engaged in scientific research in a variety of fields, created solid relationships with other foreign physicians operating in Jerusalem, and earned a place of honor in the scientific community. By virtue of these achievements and his gracious personality, the Jewish people in Jerusalem gave Chaplin the title of 'The Great English Doctor'.[33]

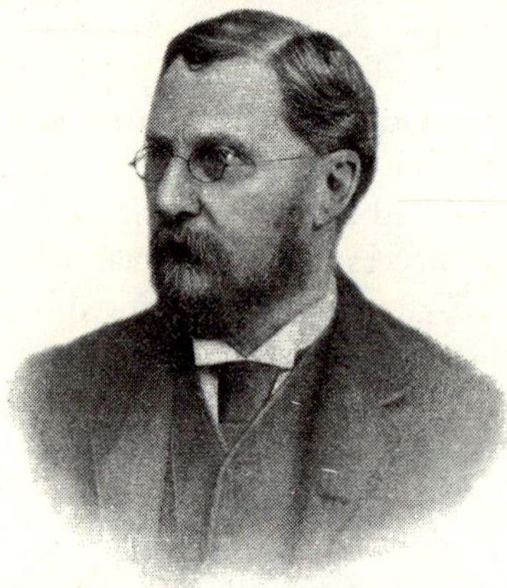

Figure 14 - Dr Thomas J. Chaplin

Thomas Chaplin was born in England in 1830. He completed his medical studies at the University of St. Andrews, and finished his medical training as a doctor at Guy's Hospital in London on January 1, 1857.[34] At the age of thirty he joined the ranks of the London Jews Society. On December 7, 1860, he replaced Dr Edward Macgowan as the director of the British medical institution in Jerusalem. Chaplin arrived in Palestine on Christmas Eve and applied himself energetically to the treatment of the Jewish patients who gathered at the gates of the hospital.

Chaplin was actively engaged in the Hospital Relief Fund established in England to collect funds and clothing for the patients. His efforts were supported by leading figures in government circles and the British nobility. Over the years as director of the hospital, Chaplin engaged in additional public activities and became a well-known figure in Jerusalem. More than once he was unable to decide which hat he should wear, that of a physician, a scientist, a public figure or a missionary. Two years after Chaplin completed his term of office in Jerusalem and having returned to London, he gave a lecture before the leaders of several British missionary societies in which he laid out in great detail his concept of a medical mission. On the basis of his personal experience in Jerusalem, he referred to the question concerning the choice before a physician who, on occasion, also serves as a missionary. In his opinion, the two functions should be separated since at that time, at the end of the nineteenth century, the demands made on a doctor's skills were too many to allow him to serve also as an active missionary. However, and here he apparently resorted to his experiences in Palestine, the medical mission must take advantage of the status of the physician in times of distress when the intervention of someone of stature and prestige was needed to confront the authorities. As he saw it, an official would find it hard to refuse the doctor's request because of his gratitude for medical treatment received in the past, and still more because of the fear that he or his colleagues might need such treatment in the future. [35] During the course of his stay in Palestine, Chaplin returned to England five times for long vacations. On one return visit he married Sophia Caroline (1833-1907), the second daughter of George William Howe Cresswell, Esq. (1800-1848). The marriage took place at St. Mark's Church, South Norwood, on November 11, 1865.[36] The couple had four children all of whom were born in Jerusalem: Emily Ada Sophia, Alfred William, Elizabeth Charlotte Maud and Janet Mabel.[37]

On January 1, 1886 Chaplin left his position after 25 years of service and returned to London. He was appointed by the London Jews Society as Inspector of Mission Stations around the world, a position that was well tailored to suit him. Within the framework of this position he paid frequent visits to Palestine and other countries in which the London Jews Society was active. On April 13, 1897, the London Jews Society inaugurated a new hospital in Jerusalem and invited its loyal doctor to the ceremonial dedication. At the height of this event, in tribute to his medical activities and his contribution to the citizens of Jerusalem, a wing of the hospital was dedicated in his name: Chaplin Ward.[38] In his speech, in the presence of the consular staff and other dignitaries, he praised the modern institution and was at pains to acknowledge all those who participated in the construction of the building. In his typically direct manner he did not forget to mention, at the end of his speech, that the new institution required additional, vitally necessary facilities, and hinted that this would incur considerable financial expense.[39]

Alongside his duties as a member of the Higher Council of the London Jews Society and responsibility for its Mission Stations around the world, Chaplin took upon himself, from 1891 onward, the direction of the medical mission of the London Jews Society in the district of Whitechapel. Towards the end of his life, especially during the supervisory visits he conducted all over the world, he suffered from various diseases, mainly malaria.[40] In spite of this, he continued his activities until October 1, 1902, when he retired and went to live at the resort of St. Leonards-on-Sea on the English Channel. On September 20, 1904, at the age of 74, Thomas Chaplin died. He was buried in the cemetery of the nearby town of Hastings.

Medical Achievements and Contribution

During the twenty-five years Chaplin spent as director of the hospital in Jerusalem, he engaged in scientific research and obtained a place of honor among international scientific circles. Among the public scientific institutions in which he was active was the Victoria Institute (an association of upper-class intellectuals, one of many functioning at that time in England). At the Institute's plenary session on May 12, 1902, his lecture 'On Some Diseases Mentioned in the Bible' was read aloud in his absence.[41] This was one of the earliest attempts to address the history of medicine in the Bible made by an early modern physician and scholar. Later on, in the early twentieth century, other scholars, such as Julius Preuss (1861-1913), who were better equipped in scientific knowledge and languages skills, published their work about medicine in the Bible and other Jewish sources.[42]

E.W. Gurney Masterman of Jerusalem commented on the lecture and subsequent discussion in a letter dated May 21, 1902.[43] His reaction, based on a decade of experience as a doctor in the country, was supportive and praised Chaplin's knowledge and analysis. Masterman noted that he valued Chaplin's work very highly, especially his comments on leprosy.

Fever research

Chaplin was known for his scientific talents in the medical field. Thus, Dr Percy Charles Edward d'Erf Wheeler (1859-1944), Chaplin's successor, eulogized: 'His clinical observations of malarial fever were of great value. His scientific contributions to the medical journal were many, the chief and best known being "The Fever of Jerusalem".[44] This article, which was published in the well-known journal *The Lancet,* gave a systematic review of the physical conditions of Jerusalem and its surroundings.[45] The article is considered by several researchers as the first scientific medical exposition originating in Palestine.[46] In the article, Chaplin applied his abilities as a doctor, researcher, and historical geographer, as well as his knowledge of the city, its environs, its climate, and its diversified population. The article began:

> Jerusalem is one of the most unhealthy cities, and fever is its principal disease. Orientals and Europeans, immigrants and natives, alike suffer, and during the sickly period of the year almost one fourth of the population become ill.[47]

This publication appeared less than four years after Chaplin arrived in Jerusalem. However, the systematic review of the physical conditions of the city, the description of the illness (the 'Syrian fever') and its symptoms, the analysis of the cases of this illness, and the conclusions he deduced from it, testify to his manifold abilities.

Leprosy

In those days, leprosy affected many in Jerusalem. Dr Gerhard Hansen (1841-1912) discovered the bacteria responsible for the disease,[48] and it was later named Hansen's Disease.[49] Chaplin conducted a detailed examination of the roots of the disease and became one of its prominent researchers. 'Of all the diseases which afflict humanity, leprosy is one of the most terrible', he wrote about the subject, including a detailed description of leprosy in his book 'On Some Diseases Mentioned in the Bible'.[50] He added a learned discourse on the biblical 'tzara'ath' and other skin diseases.[51] Dr Wheeler, Chaplin's successor as head of the English Mission Hospital wrote: 'He made a careful and systematic examination of each leper in Jerusalem and Ramleh, and was at that time one of the authorities on leprosy'.[52]

Chaplin guided the Baroness Augusta Keffenbrinck-Ascheraden (1835-1889) and her husband Baron Wilhelm Friedrich (1823-1896) of Germany, in Jerusalem in 1865. Thereafter the couple donated money for a lepers' sanatorium in Jerusalem. Chaplin became a member of the directorate of the German institution (*Jesus Hilfe* - The Help of Jesus) and later was appointed the chief physician there until his departure from Jerusalem early in 1886.

Researchers attempting to assess the quality of the treatment may analyze the reports and descriptions of the patients, their conditions and the treatment which the lepers in the hospital were getting, along with the fact that Chaplin was consulting known experts such as Prof. Heinrich Haesser (1811-1884) of Breslau in Germany. Several researchers have concluded that the treatment in the hospital was humane and modern.[53]

Through Chaplin's dedicated work on leprosy, and by his efforts in learning, healing and building a hospital for the lepers in the Holy Land, he eased the suffering of the lepers and acted to alleviate the deep social and moral stigma that confronted victims for centuries. By doing so, Chaplin fulfilled Titus Tobler's wishes by using his talents in both administration and public relations.

Eye diseases

Chaplin was involved in erecting another hospital in Jerusalem to ease eye diseases, one of the most widespread afflictions in Palestine. Combining his duties as a physician with his goal of serving the public at large, Chaplin served as an Honorary Associate of the Council of the Order of St. John of Jerusalem. In the beginning of the 1880s he took part in an important initiative to establish the Ophthalmic Hospital in Jerusalem.[54]

Climatology

In the spring of 1863, during a tour of the country, Dr Keith Johnston (1804-1871), General Secretary of the Scottish Meteorological Society, met Chaplin in Jerusalem and reached an agreement with him to carry out climate measurements. The Scottish society supplied the instruments, including barometers and thermometers. After more than three years of observations, a preliminary article was published in the *Journal of the Scottish Meteorological Society* with a parallel paper in the *Palestine Exploration Fund Quarterly Statement.*

The report provided daily measurements of barometric pressure, temperature, and condensation in Jerusalem, comparisons with other cities in the Middle East, and analyses.[55] Chaplin later became a full-fledged member of the Scottish meteorological society and wrote a monograph on the climate of Jerusalem which was published in 1883 in three scientific forums: in the journal of the German society for the research of Palestine– *Zeitschrift des Deutschen Palästina-Vereins* (*ZDPV*), in the *PEFQS*, and in the *Journal of the Scottish Meteorological Society.* The monograph presented detailed climate observations and summarized the daily condensation measurements in Jerusalem, which serves till today as a basis for the climate research of nineteenth century Palestine.[56]

Interestingly, Chaplin was not the first to conduct climate observation in the Holy Land in the nineteenth century. That honor belongs to his predecessor Dr Edward Macgowan. Macgowan started taking measurements in 1846 at the old hospital in Jerusalem, though he never published his findings. Chaplin continued Macgowan's activities and, by publishing his findings, laid the foundation on which climatologists could compare their findings until the present day.[57]

Linguistics

Chaplin showed proficiency and mastered Hebrew, Arabic, Spanish, German, and Yiddish.[58] He used his talents in linguistic research and in the art of translation, by translating from Hebrew into English the Mishnaic tractates describing the Temple and its rites - *Yoma*, *Tamid*, and *Middoth* – along with the commentary of Rabbi Obadiah di Bertinoro (fifteenth-sixteenth century).[59] Chaplin also translated the treatise *Beth Habehira* by Maimonides (1138-1204), the famous Jewish rabbi and scholar,[60] and served as a member of the Committee of the British and Foreign Bible Society. In that capacity, he translated into Yiddish the *Gospel According to Saint Matthew*. However, while his translations were important during his time, they have not left any significant mark in present times.

Archeology

Like many other Europeans in Palestine in the nineteenth century, Chaplin engaged in archaeological excavations. He reported his findings to the Palestine Exploration Fund (PEF). However, his main contribution to research of the Land of Israel seems to have been his editorship for a dozen years of the *PEFQS* in which he published many articles. His research also appeared in the *Survey of Western Palestine*. The *Survey* was written by Charles Warren and Claude Reignier Conder (1848-1910), members of the PEF and among the greatest researchers in nineteenth century Palestine.[61]

For example, Chaplin provided the following reports:

- In 1871 Chaplin visited the Hummam esh-Shefa, one of the five baths in Jerusalem, also known as the Bath of Salvation, which is situated near the Cotton Market on the western side of the Temple Mount. He wrote a report containing a detailed description of the site, which was published in the *PEFQS* and in the *Survey of Western Palestine*.[62]
- In August 1873, Chaplin published a report on the discovery of Cufic inscriptions on the roof of the Dome of the Rock building[63] and on discoveries of a burial cave in Jerusalem: 'More than 20 mortuary chests discovered at rock tombs in Mount of Offence…' In this scholarly report he uses cautious language with regard to his conclusions: 'The reasons which lead me to think it possible… are these…' and he then details four explanations for his caution. In one of them his modesty is expressed: 'at least to my unprofessional eye...'.[64] His detailed

report is still used by archeologists today and is considered professional and important.[65]

- Five days after filing his report on the Dome of the Rock, he sent an additional letter on the subject with new details, apologizing for having forgotten to report earlier. In this letter he shows his knowledge of Islamic history, and one sentence reveals the conflict between his vocation as a physician and his avocation as a researcher of Jerusalem and the Land of Israel: 'it is only with great effort that I can give any time to these things at this sickly period of the year'.[66]
- Chaplin was an active participant in the discovery and decipherment of the Siloam inscription dating from the First Temple period. The inscription describes the work of those excavating a tunnel to carry water from the Gihon Spring, which was then outside the walls of Jerusalem, to the Siloam Pool within the walls of first Temple Period Jerusalem.[67]

Even when Chaplin was unable to participate in research expeditions in Palestine and neighboring countries because of his commitments at the hospital, he supported and greatly assisted other researchers. For example, Charles Conder reported that Chaplin donated £25 for lowering the water level in the Siloam Pool tunnel, thus exposing the inscription. In this case, even though Chaplin was unable to provide scientific assistance, he supported the project financially and in spirit. Charles Warren, mentioned above as a founder of the Palestine Exploration Fund, made sure to note in a report sent from Transjordan in August 1867 that 'I have received much assistance from the British residents here, especially from Dr Brewer, Dr Barclay and Dr Chaplin, which I should like you to mention if you will write again to the papers'.[68]

Reading Chaplin's reports, one can clearly feel his love for archeological experiences. Nevertheless, Chaplin's archeological endeavours were limited to his off-duty time, which was rare in the sickly atmosphere of nineteenth century Jerusalem. Therefore, although his archeological contribution was seriously regarded in his time, it did not leave much impact on modern day archeology.[69]

Historical Geography

Chaplin applied his knowledge and expertise in ancient sources to his research in the field of historical geography. His 1888 article 'The Site of Ebenezer' identified Even ha-Ezer – the site of the decisive battle between the Philistines and the Israelites – with the village of Beit Iksa near Jerusalem. In his article Chaplin adduced sound reasons for his identification, utilizing various scientific techniques and demonstrating his thorough familiarity with historical sources such as the writings of Josephus Flavius, the Church Father Eusebius (260-340) and, of course, the Bible.[70] His scholarly opinion notwithstanding, Chaplin's name is neither mentioned nor known among geographer-historians and researchers dealing with biblical times and events.[71]

International Politics and Vision of the Jews' Future

In addition to being a renowned doctor and a skilled scientist, Chaplin was an ardent religious missionary and an educated scholar. He had firm convictions about the role of the British Mission and its potential to influence the future of the Jewish people. In May 1898, Chaplin gave a speech and set forth his views before the plenum of the London Jews Society at its annual meeting. He began by referring to the nineteenth century and opining that in all the recorded annals of the nations there had never been a similar period in human history in which such significant changes had taken place. The development of scientific skills, the inculcation of the values of freedom, and the widening use of fast communication methods among the various political powers had changed the face of the world and the course of human life. In Chaplin's opinion, no nation was more influenced by these surprising developments than the Jewish people, because their members were well established in most of the enterprises associated with science, art, trade and industry, and were closely linked with most of the cultural circles. Chaplin believed that young Jews everywhere, even in the strongholds of rabbinical Judaism, eagerly yearned for contact with the outside world. He believed that Jews sought to break through barriers of isolation and make use of the power inherent within the Jewish character in order to take an active part in the social and intellectual struggles of their day.

However, aware as he was of the situation of the Jewish people, Chaplin also knew of the new factor that characterized his time - the revival of hatred towards the Jews and of anti-Semitic persecution in Eastern Europe. For the greater part of human history Jews were subject to scorn and persecution, but it might have been expected that at the time when there was free and enlightened social development the persecution of the Jews would cease. That, of course, was not the case. Chaplin addressed this as follows:

> Yet not only Russia, with its despotic methods of government, but Austria, Germany, Romania, and even enlightened and humanitarian France have raised their voices, and even lifted their hands, against this long-suffering and afflicted race. In Algiers recently I saw 'liberty, equality, fraternity' inscribed on the walls of public buildings within sight of Jewish shops which had been pillaged, wrecked and burned. Why is this? What is the cause that, even under the most civilized governments, outrages of this kind take place?[72]

As a believing missionary, Chaplin attributed this internal contradiction to the will of God. In his view, the Almighty must have decreed that the Jewish people would not find permanent security anywhere in the world until it inhabited the land that God had given to its forefathers.

Chaplin visited Jerusalem in 1897 to participate in the festivities marking the inauguration of the new hospital of the London Jews Society, and saw with his own eyes the development of the Jewish settlements. He wrote:

> It is a delight to visit the agricultural settlements in the Holy Land, with their beautiful gardens of palm-trees and flowering shrubs, their vineyards, and cornfields, and comfortable houses, in such strong contrast to the poverty and squalor of the native villages around. But whether these settlements have been established on a sound basis, whether they spring from a spontaneous impulse of the Jewish people, or are merely charitable efforts of Jewish philanthropists doomed to fail when extraneous support is withdrawn, it is yet too early to

> know. For my own part, I am not able to contemplate this remarkable movement without feeling that the hand of God is in it. For more than thirty years I have watched with keenest interest the continuous, and at times rapid influx of Jews into the Holy Land, the spread of education among them there, their awakening to a more active intellectual life, their readiness to learn mechanical trades whereby to gain a livelihood, their gradual, though tardy, realization of the truth that to work is as much man's duty as to pray. I cannot help thinking that this movement will go on, and perhaps eventually result in changes of a very important character.[73]

When Thomas Chaplin gave his speech in London in May 1898, it was only nine months after the gathering of the First Zionist Congress in Basle in which the institutions of the Zionist movement were established. The Congress, in which some of the London Jews Society members participated as observers, left a deep impression on the missionaries who saw this gathering as a sign of the coming redemption. The journal of the London Jews Society followed the events with great interest, and printed in full the speeches of the leaders of the Zionist movement, Theodor Herzl (1860-1904), Max Nordau (1849-1923), and others.

It was this strong impression that prompted Chaplin to refer in his speech to the phenomenon of national awakening among the Jewish people and to appraise its chances. Zionism 'was sprouting' and looking forward to reestablishing a Jewish state in the Holy Land. Many such associations actively encouraged the flourishing new Jewish settlements in Palestine, investing considerable sums for this purpose. Significant progress was evident.

When Chaplin died in 1904, he was eulogized in the *Palestine Exploration Fund Quarterly Statement* as follows:

> The Palestine Exploration Fund has lost a staunch supporter and tried friend in the late Dr Chaplin… From the foundation of the Fund, Dr Chaplin took a keen interest in its work, and the success that attended its operation in the field during the first twenty-one years of its existence was largely due to his

> unreserved kindness and thoughtful care...He tended the explorers when sick, gave them the best advice in sanitary matters, and unreservedly placed at their disposal his great knowledge of Jerusalem and the Holy Land, and of the people amongst whom he lived and laboured for twenty-five years.[74]

It is a complex task to portray the character of a person who died nearly a century ago. Doing so can be frustrating when the subject is seen to be outstanding and prolific, while the extant written material about him is so meager. Concerning himself, Thomas Chaplin stated: 'I believe it is a very good rule to do one's work and let other people talk about it'.[75] Chaplin published the fruits of his research in a variety of subjects, delivered memorable lectures, but left others to speak his praise during his lifetime and after his death. During his long and full life he was active in many fields and left an indelible imprint on his patients, who admired him as a man and as a physician. He also left his mark on his fellow researchers of the Holy Land, whom he attended when they fell ill, supported in their work, and joined in their explorations and in the many discoveries they made. For many years, enthusiastic supporters of Palestine and its research read Chaplin's scholarly articles, and doctors around the world learnt from him about the medical problems and diseases of Jerusalem.

A review of his deeds in the Holy Land reveals the diversity of his published works and achievements:

A. His medical work improved the condition of Jerusalem and its inhabitants' health for a quarter of a century. His medical research and original publications were foundations for further study and lead to international progress in several medical fields. The hospitals and medical institutions that were built through his efforts and initiative were important to the city for many years and are part of the city's landscape even now (although no longer serving as medical institutions).

B. Chaplin's missionary work cannot be considered as a great success. He used his off-duty time for research and writing and not for religious and missionary activities, as other physicians did (Dr Wheeler for example).

C. Chaplin's public relations and his administrative abilities were unique and helped him and the mission to develop projects and therefore to improve medicine in Jerusalem. As a result, he increased the influence of the mission and the British people in the Holy Land at a time of competition between the European Powers.

D. Because Chaplin devoted most of his off-duty time to research of the Holy Land in general and Jerusalem in particular, the impact of his findings and publications as an archeologist, linguist and historical geographer were minor. Working in these fields, as in others, takes learned skills, full devotion and consistency – and a physician and head of a medical mission, notwithstanding his considerable talent, could hardly excel in those other areas. We should bear in mind that in the nineteenth century the Holy Land and Jerusalem were flooded with European archeologists and researchers, most of whom were better skilled than Chaplin and devoted full time to their work. Of all the many reports he wrote, only two or three are still known and in use today. In contrast – Chaplin's climatological observations are of great importance because he was the first to publish scientific observations in the Holy Land in general and in Jerusalem in particular.

His talents as a researcher were of value first and foremost to the London Jews Society. The Mission benefited from his services as an excellent doctor and from his good relations and wide-ranging contacts among the elite in Jerusalem. It likewise benefited from his organizational and management skills as director of its medical institution, from his mastery of languages, and from his abilities as initiator of the construction of various medical facilities. Finally, it profited from his experience and his service as supervisor and controller of the Mission's stations around the world, in the closing years of his professional career. Chaplin did not hesitate to take advantage of his social contacts, his public office, and his diverse talents to advance and develop the voluntary medical services in Jerusalem, as demonstrated by his efforts to set up the sanatorium for lepers and the hospital for eye diseases in the city.

Dr Percy Charles Edward d'Erf Wheeler (1859-1944)

Percy Charles Edward d'Erf Wheeler was born in December 14, 1859, the firstborn son of Captain d'Erf Wheeler, Chief of Police in Mauritius. Percy and his two brothers were raised in India by an aunt. From childhood Wheeler wanted to become a medical missionary, and eventually began his training at the Madras Medical College. Upon returning to England, he studied at St. Thomas's Hospital where he passed his primary examinations in anatomy and physiology in the spring of 1884 as an outstanding student.[76] That year, his long-standing dream came true when he joined the London Jews Society.[77]

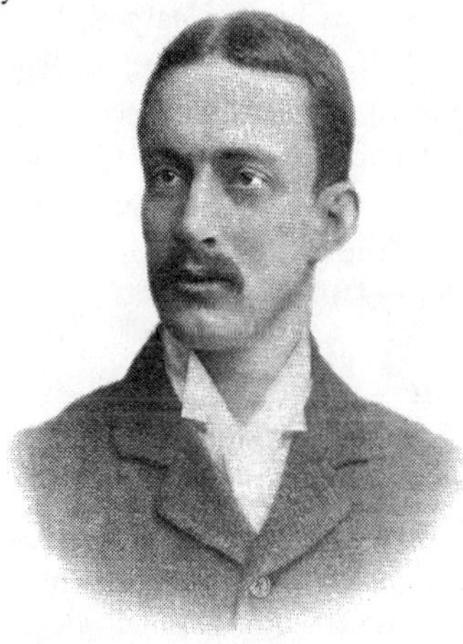

Figure 15 - Dr Percy Charles Edward d'Erf Wheeler

When Wheeler arrived in Jerusalem in 1885, the British hospital was the jewel in the crown of the missionary endeavour and medical work of the London Jews Society in Palestine.[78] However it was located in a modest building inside the city walls. The need for a new hospital in Jerusalem arose as early as the mid-1870s because of the dilapidated state of the old hospital building and the increasing rate of occupancy during that period. The initial step to build the new hospital was taken only at the end of 1889, through the generosity of an English woman who anonymously donated £1,000 to the building fund.[79] Planning for the new hospital was entrusted to British architect, Beresford Pite, who completed the assignment at the end of 1891.[80] On April 13, 1897, the London Jews Society inaugurated its new Hospital for the Jews in Jerusalem, its flagship in Palestine and the institution in which most of the funds and attention were invested.[81]

On July 5, 1893, Wheeler married Grace Blyth (b. 1872), the second daughter of Reverend George Francis Popham Blyth (1832-1914), Anglican Bishop of Jerusalem and the East, at Christ Church in Jerusalem.[82] They had a daughter and three sons; the older two sons died in the First World War.[83]

Wheeler's academic credentials were outstanding. In November 1891 he was informed that he had passed the final examination for the FRCS.[84] In 1892, he was awarded a degree in Medicine and Surgery with honours.[85] In 1906, he became a Fellow of the Royal Institute of Public Health in London.[86] He was nominated Honorary Local Secretary for the Palestine Exploration Fund (PEF) in Jerusalem, succeeding the late Archdeacon T.E. Dowling. He held this post from 1896 until 1909.

On several occasions, the London Jews Society sent Wheeler to England to give lectures and raise fund. His tours in 1891 and 1897 raised money for the new hospital in Jerusalem.[87] The texts of his lectures in England and Ireland provide information on his work as a physician and a missionary and attest to his affection for the Jewish People, especially since he served in the Holy Land at the time of its rebuilding by the Jews. His enthusiastic descriptions of the new Jewish settlements are historically accurate, sincere, and vivid.[88]

His attitude toward the Jews of Jerusalem and the importance he ascribed to the missionaries' medical initiatives are well reflected in his writings. He described Jewish frustration and the remedies the missionaries were ready to provide:

> For nineteen centuries the Jews were persecuted and persecuted and persecuted. They say 'There is no use to talking to us. You tell us that God is holy and that Christ is love, where is the love? ' Now we tell them, 'Yes, that is what we come out here for – to show you that Christ loves you and

> that we love you in practical way'. You have no idea of the power that the hospital has over them. When they come to us to relieve them, and they find we do all we can for them, they are so grateful.[89]

Wheeler's descriptions helped the Society to publicize what was required and to raise the necessary funds to develop additional medical institutions in the Holy Land.[90]

Another way of presenting the work at the Jerusalem hospital was by publishing pictures in the London Jews Society's Journal, *The Jewish Missionary Intelligence* (JMI). In the June, 1907, issue, four pictures show several patients in different rooms of the new hospital's wards; the captions describe the facilities and hard work of the medical staff, and the journal recognized the contributors of the Society and the help they provided for the sick and needy at the Holy City. The article concludes with a quote from Wheeler:

> This is the work that is so potent, and hoping to destroy prejudices against Christianity. It wins the heart of the most bigoted Jew – for he is still human – and conquers where everything else fails. Those four cases [shown in the pictures] are in themselves lessons to both Jews and Christians, and these are a few amongst many we have during the year ...[91]

The medical activities in Jerusalem were not limited to the hospital or the dispensary; Wheeler and his fellow physicians paid home visits to their Jewish patients as well.[92] In addition, in 1896, immediately after the Society inaugurated its new hospital outside the Old City of Jerusalem, the old hospital within the walls continued to function as a dispensary for the inhabitants of the Jewish quarter. In January 1900, Dr Ernest William Gurney Masterman, who had served since December 1892 under Wheeler, became the director of the old hospital. Masterman also practiced several days a week in a clinic in the village of Siloam near Jerusalem, treating the recently immigrated Yemenite Jews.[93]

In October 1909, Wheeler, the senior medical missionary of the London Jews Society in Jerusalem since 1885, retired after twenty-four years of 'most active and strenuous service'.[94] He was succeeded by Dr Masterman.[95] In 1910, after his return to England,

Wheeler undertook the task of working among the Jews of North London and was appointed 'Honorary Consulting Physician to the Society'.[96]

On March 30, 1910, Wheeler received a moving letter from his mostly Christian friends and colleagues in Jerusalem and London entitled 'Testimonial to Dr d'Erf Wheeler': the content sheds light on their view of Wheeler's personality and character:

> On the occasion of his leaving Jerusalem after twenty-four years of excited service as Head of the Medical Mission of the London Jews Society for Promoting Christianity amongst the Jews, the friends of Dr Percy d'Erf Wheeler, in Palestine and at home, desire to show their sincere regard for him, and their high appreciation of his work. They therefore beg his acceptance of this address and the accompanying purse of money. They pray that the blessing of God may rest upon him and his, and trust that he may still be granted many years of happy life and service.

The testimonial was signed by the British Consul in Jerusalem, the Anglican Bishop in Jerusalem and dozens of friends in England and Palestine.[97]

Wheeler's reply, published in the London Jews Society's journal, tell us more about how the physician was spending his time:

> A few days ago I received an address beautifully illuminated, and accompanied by your generous gift of money. I wish it were in my power to write to each one of you, to tell you how deeply touched I am by your thought of me. But I must content myself with these few words which I am sending to the magazine to thank you, one and all, most warmly for such a generous and practical appreciation of my service in Jerusalem... I always look back with happy remembrances on the years I spent in Jerusalem ... My time is so fully occupied now in my new work, that very little is left me for correspondence... [98]

In 1913 Dr Wheeler was nominated by the Royal Society of Medicine to a small Reference Committee formed at the request of the Privy Council. In 1915, during the First World War, he joined the Royal Army Medical Corps (RAMC) and served in Egypt. For his work later at Canterbury and Shoreham, he received the Army Council's thanks for 'his excellent work'.

During the First World War, the British hospitals in Palestine were taken over by the Turkish military and the British doctors returned home. After the war, in September 1919, Wheeler left England for Palestine with his wife and daughter. In October 1919, after renovations, he reopened one of the hospital wards in Jerusalem.[99] His successor in years to come, Dr H J Orr-Ewing, described in the Society's journal the process of resuming medical work after the war, referring to the role assumed by Wheeler: 'No one could have reopened the work in such a glorious way ... The magic of his [Wheeler's] name was still a mighty force in Jerusalem, and his return was the sign to the Jews that the Hospital really was to reopen as before'.[100]

Wheeler left the Holy Land in 1921 and continued to work among the Jews in East London until 1937. He died on November 28, 1944.

Dr Percy Charles Edward d'Erf Wheeler dedicated the many years he served in Palestine in promoting the medical condition of the Jews as a means of missionary work. To this end he practised as a physician and made the work undertaken by his staff common knowledge in England by presenting lectures and publishing articles in the Society's journal for the purpose of fund raising. The most significant of his achievements was his leading role in the founding of the new English Mission Hospital for the Jews in Jerusalem. He was known especially for procuring the endowment of most of the beds and cots and for ensuring medical staff salaries.

Wheeler's detailed reports on the work in the Mission hospital in Jerusalem from 1907 to 1909 reveal that he treated some 500 in-patients and 4,400 out-patients, making 1,500 home visits, applying 6,000 dressings, writing 9000 prescriptions and having 20,000 receipts. The report indicates how hard and important was the work undertaken by the physicians, nurses, and other staff of the hospital and dispensary.[101]

Unlike other European physicians serving in Palestine, including Dr Chaplin who preceded him[102] and Dr Masterman who succeeded him,[103] Wheeler did not engage in scientific work or publish scientific articles or books. Nevertheless, his knowledge of Jewish history, character and customs was unique and helpful. Full of love for the opportunity the people of Israel afforded him and his medical practice, he considered the twenty-four years he spent in Jerusalem as 'the happiest of his life'.[104]

Dr Ernest William Gurney Masterman (1867-1943)

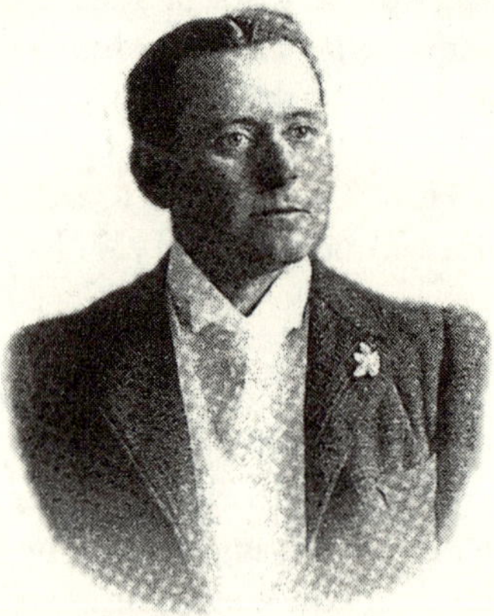

Figure 16 - Dr Ernest William Gurney Masterman

Ernest Masterman was born on January 2, 1867, in Rotherfield Hall, Sussex. He was the eldest son of Thomas William Masterman (d. c.1893) and Margaret Hanson Gurney. One of his brothers was the Right Hon. Charles Frederick Gurney Masterman.[105] Ernest was educated at Clifton College and at Monkton Combe School. He was attracted to the vocation of a medical missionary, in preparation for which he studied first at Edinburgh University in 1884, where he became acquainted with C.T. Studd (1860-1931), the well-known evangelist. Owing to family circumstances his studies were interrupted, and for a time he took up the position of schoolmaster. In 1887 he entered St. Bartholomew's Hospital in London, where he was Brackenbury surgical scholar, qualifying in 1891. In that same year he became a member of the Royal College of Surgeons of England (MRCS) and Licentiate of the Royal College of Physicians of London (LRCP). A year later Masterman earned the higher surgical qualification of a Fellow of the Royal College of Surgeons of England (FRCS). In 1899 he received the Diploma in Public Health (DPH) from the University of Cambridge and in 1909 he was awarded the degree of Doctor of Medicine (MD) by the University of Durham.[106]

In 1892, Masterman attained his goal and was appointed Assistant Medical Officer at the English Mission Hospital in Jerusalem. In October of that year, Masterman left England, and en route to Jerusalem, he stayed for a while in Constantinople to obtain the Turkish diploma needed to practice medicine in the Ottoman Empire. He reached Jerusalem in December 1892 and took up his post under Dr Percy d'Erf Wheeler, director of the English Mission Hospital.

In May 1893, Masterman conducted a tour of inspection to the Galilean city of Safed in northern Palestine with Arthur Hastings Kelk, head of the London Mission in the Holy Land. A month later he replaced Alexander Robert Iliewitz (1815-1895), the aged missionary who had been serving at the modest Safed Mission of the London Jews Society and was now returning to Jerusalem. Immediately upon Masterman's arrival, he sent London his impressions of the importance of Safed as a mission station and of the pressing need to strengthen that post by establishing a proper hospital for the inhabitants in the city. As a result, Dr Walter Henry Anderson was sent to Safed to establish a new hospital to be inaugurated in May 31, 1904.

On May 23, 1894 Masterman married Louisa Nazarina Zeller (1873-1908) at Christ Church in Jerusalem. She was the sixth daughter of the German missionary Johannes Zeller (1830-1902) and Hanna Maria-Sophie (1838-1922), daughter of the second Protestant bishop in Jerusalem, Samuel Gobat (1799-1879).[107] Louisa bore five children but died young, on April 27, 1908, and was buried in the Protestant cemetery on Mount Zion.[108] On August 8, 1909, Masterman was married again, to Johanna Zeller, his late wife's sister at St. John's Church in Tunbridge Wells, England.

In mid-1895, Masterman was sent to Damascus on behalf of the Eustace Maxwell Memorial Fund.[109] After practicing surgery at the medical institute there for one year, he returned to Jerusalem. By that time, the London Jews Society had inaugurated its new hospital outside the Old City of Jerusalem. The old hospital within the walls operated as a dispensary for the inhabitants of the Jewish quarter. From January 1900, Masterman served as the director of this modest institution, and parallel to this main practice, he worked in another missionary medical institution. During the 1880s, thousands of Yemenite Jews immigrated to the Holy Land and settled in Jerusalem. The Jewish community of the city could not finance their absorption and refused to adopt the new immigrants. Some of the Yemenite newcomers, with the help of Protestant missionaries, settled in Siloam (Kfar Ha-Shiloah), an Arab village south of the Old City. The London Jews Society began to make regular visits there and offered the residents medical assistance. In 1900, when the number of the Yemenite Jews reached 3,500, Masterman obtained a house to use for a clinic in Siloam and visited there several times a week.[110]

In the autumn of 1909, in consideration of the 18 years he had spent serving as physician, deputy to the general director of the hospital, and head of the dispensary in Jerusalem, Masterman was appointed to succeed Dr D'Erf Wheeler as head of all medical services of the London Jews Society in the Holy Land. He held this position until the outbreak of the First World War, when, as a national of a coalition state at war with Turkey, he was forced to leave Palestine.

Masterman returned to England in 1914, and after a spell at the Military Hospital in Coventry, he became resident superintendent of St. Giles Hospital in Camberwell, London, and held this position until he reached the statutory retirement age in 1934. Having no desire for a life of idleness, he offered his medical services and his knowledge of Palestine to the Church Missionary Society, an offer that was readily accepted.[111] Masterman was commissioned to establish and equip a hospital at Es-Salt in Trans-Jordan, and within two years he accomplished the task. In 1938, at the age of 71 he was appointed Medical Superintendent of the General Hospitals in Palestine, and in 1939 he was appointed medical adviser for the Near East to the Church Missionary Society.[112]

Masterman's health began to fail, and he died in Jerusalem on March 29, 1943 in the presence of his second wife and other family members. He was buried at the Protestant cemetery on Mount Zion.

For almost forty-five years Ernest William Gurney Masterman held a variety of positions in Jerusalem, besides serving as a physician at the English Mission Hospital for the Jews in Jerusalem.[113] In the midst of the turbulence of the Second World War, the Palestine Exploration Fund in its *Quarterly Statement* of 1943 mourned the loss of Masterman in these words: 'By the death of Dr. Masterman, the Palestine Exploration Fund has lost one who, for almost a century, had found time in a strenuous professional life to further its interests and its undertakings in every possible way'.[114]

Researcher of the Holy Land

Masterman constantly pursued knowledge and research, a fact that is best described in an obituary published in the *Palestine Exploration Quarterly*:

> From the time of his first arrival in Jerusalem he became a whole-hearted student of 'Palestinology' in all its branches. Nothing came amiss – history, geography, and antiquities: anthropology, physical and social: geology, zoology, botany, climatology, and the possibilities of future development under the happier circumstances inaugurated by the revolution which swept the last of the sultans from his throne… his first contribution to the Quarterly Statement appeared in 1896, and was followed by stream of others, touching on many aspects of the Fund's work...[115]

Besides his literary contributions to its publications, Masterman took part in the activities of the Palestine Exploration Fund. He was a frequent and ever-welcome visitor to the Fund's excavations, inspecting every new discovery, encouraging the directors, entering the most difficult caves and tunnels, and giving medical care to the staff and employees. In 1910 he succeeded Dr Wheeler as Honorary Secretary of the Fund in Jerusalem. When he returned to London in 1914 because of the outbreak of the war, he succeeded the deceased J.D. Crace as Honorary General Secretary of the fund, an office he held until his return to Palestine. In 1934, he assumed the task of Honorary Secretary in Jerusalem.[116]

Due to the knowledge he had accumulated while researching the Holy Land, Masterman was selected to be co-editor of the famous Cook's handbook for Palestine and Syria.[117] The publishers of those handbooks, like the well known Baedeker and others, sought local scholars to write about the parts that they probably knew best. This commission confirms him as an expert at the forefront of knowledge of the Holy Land.

Jerusalem studies and politics (local and international)

Masterman, who spent more than twenty years researching and accumulating data, became an expert on the city of Jerusalem. In his article 'Jerusalem outside the walls'[118] he describes the important and historical process whereby the Jewish community in Jerusalem began to leave the Jewish quarter and settle outside the walls of the Old City, a move that began in the 1860s and reached its peak during the last two decades of the nineteenth century. The innovation of this article is that while other authors of the period wrote mainly about Jerusalem's holy sites, Masterman sensed the importance of describing the new Jewish neighbourhoods, rarely visited then, but which reshaped the new part of the city. His descriptions are based above all on his deep understanding and wide knowledge of the different communities in the city. In 1895 he wrote:

> In modern warfare such buildings as these could be of little real use for defensive purposes, so that the accusation sometimes brought against these nations, especially against Russia, that in building these structures, they have been preparing for a warlike occupation of the country is, I believe, quite without any support. In the event of Moslem rising which could not be speedily suppressed by the military, these massive structures would undoubtedly greatly help the

> Russians and Latin Christians to defend themselves for a time, and it is quite possible that during a European war with Turkey they might be called into such a use.[119]

His deep acquaintance with the inner life in the city and the different segments of its population, together with his understanding of global politics poised for the First World War, made him an authority on contemporary Palestine. In a lecture delivered in London before the Committee of the London Jews Society in 1909, he guided his audience deep into the internal politics of the Ottoman Empire with its implications for the Jews in the Holy Land, and hence for future missionary efforts by the Society's members:

> Almost all the people I have met [in England…] have asked about the new political outlook in Palestine, and although it is not directly a missionary subject it has a very great bearing upon our work. There were remarkable scenes when the new Constitution was sprung upon the people, many went off their heads with joy. They understood it meant liberty, and thought they were now going to do what they liked. The Jews naturally expected the fulfillment of their national hopes and that they would possess Palestine. But the 'Young Turkey' party has a strong national feeling and will not allow a single bit of ground to pass into independent hands. At the same time it will immensely facilitate the acquiring of land in Palestine, and the settling there, in greater numbers, of Jewish colonists; and there is evidence that this will lead to a greater influx of Jews.[120]

Because of his unique knowledge of Jerusalem's residents and his experience working among the Jews as physician and missionary, his descriptions are accurate and well prepared. Yet Masterman preferred to illumine the less romantic corners of the city and its inhabitants, especially the Jews. Therefore, parallel with his descriptions of the new Jewish neighborhoods outside the walls he dealt with the 'new secular Jews' of the Holy Land. In a speech to the annual meeting of the London Jews Society on the eve of the outbreak of the war he said:

> You see in that city to-day representatives of every nation under heaven. I have good authority for saying that you hear spoken in Jerusalem every day fifty languages and dialects, and the majority of them are spoken amongst the Jews. They are not united by one religion. … There is an increasing number of those who are attracted by atheism, scepticism [sic.], and materialism. They have no serious outlook upon life, and do not hold fast to the national idea. But all the Jews in Jerusalem are, with very few exceptions, united together in this one thing. They may believe or not believe what they like, but they must not be Christians.[121]

A scientist first and foremost, Masterman felt the need to shed the typical romantic aura that encompassed the holy city. He was not affected by the emotional descriptions by visitors to the city, which were meant for a European audience of Christian believers. He was a functionary of a British mission working among the Jewish people, and he painted that activity in dull colors:

> Some may say … it is so very romantic, and all that kind of thing, but if you knew our work when we settle to it, you would know it is a daily round of common duties. There is nothing specially romantic in living in Jerusalem, or working among the Jews.[122]

Masterman's profound knowledge of the country, its topography, climate, history, and other aspects were used by him to advantage in a unique book on the First World War in Palestine entitled *The Deliverance of Jerusalem.* This book, which was published in 1918 soon after the armistice,[123] gives an account of the war in Palestine, with detailed descriptions of each of the big cities and the most important areas known to the public. After setting forth the story of the battlefields around Jerusalem and an account of the modern city, Masterman wrote a chapter on his view of the future of Palestine.

In addition, his grasp of international politics, the nature and features of the land and the forces operating on it were presented in a paper read at a meeting of the Geographical Society on March 19,

1917, and later published in the Society's journal. The detailed description of Palestine, its borders, and Christian, Jewish and Muslim interests in its future, with his perception of the 'thorny problem' that all this meant for the future, was merely the introduction. Masterman then detailed the composition of the country's contemporary population, history, and inhabitants, and the new colonization process of the Christians (Americans and Germans) and the Jewish Zionist movement. He also mentioned the harsh geographical and climatic conditions of the different zones and the prevalent diseases, followed by a summary of the few natural resources and the antiquated agriculture. Masterman received praise from his listeners for his excellent paper, and Prof. Leonard King (1869-1919), chairman of the Palestine Exploration Fund, summed it up nicely:

> I think we have all been struck by the very impartial way in which Dr. Masterman has treated what must be regarded as a thorny question… on this and similar questions I think no one is better qualified than Dr. Masterman to offer advice… he has acted as local secretary of the P.E.F and I should like to take this opportunity, on behalf of the society, of saying how much we are indebted to him for all he has done for the Fund during his residence in Palestine. After the war I hope we shall again have the benefit of his advice.[124]

Geography and hydrology

An example of an inter-disciplinary study, reflecting knowledge and understanding of various fields such as the history and archaeology of Jerusalem, the city's topography, the existing infrastructure, and modern projects, emerges from an early publication on the water supply for Jerusalem.[125] One of the important non-medical research projects in which Masterman had a key role was the long-term measurement of the level of the Dead Sea. A reference to this is made in his obituary:

> A question having arisen as to whether the level of the Dead Sea is changing, Dr. Masterman determined to test it. He went down to Jericho with a stonemason, and thence along the rugged western shore of the Dead Sea, till, at 'Ain Feshkhah'

> he found a precipitous rock rising from the water. The mason was then directed to cut a mark at the convenient height from the surface of the water; and thereafter Dr. Masterman undertook the tiresome ride to the spot, once a month, in order to record the height of the water in reference to the mark. These observations were published in the Quarterly Statements from 1902 to 1913; although the local Bedouin, themselves unseen, had noticed these periodical visits, and being suspicious of their uncomprehended purpose, had destroyed the reference mark.'[126]

This description of an aspect of Masterman's scientific investigations tells us something about the way he operated. On those monthly trips, he also explored other issues in the same geographic zone, including visits to archaeological sites such as Khirbet Qumran and to fresh water springs such as Ein Feshkhah. He subsequently recorded his observations from these visits.[127]

Ethnography, biology and sociology

Masterman exploited his time in the Galilean city of Safed by taking many scientific tours and he conducted diverse research. His periodic articles appearing in different journals ultimately yielded a book named *Studies in Galilee.*[128] One of the issues that he researched on his travels to the Sea of Galilee was fishery and the fishermen, according to the accounts in the Bible and especially in the New Testament. In this article Masterman describes the different fish species of the lake, their names in several languages, the management and taxation of the fisheries business by the Ottoman authorities, their market (mainly the members of the Jewish community in Safed), and the wide range of fishing methods.[129]

In a joint series of studies, Masterman and Robert Alexander Stewart Macalister (1870-1950) reviewed the wide variety of subjects dealt with themselves and many other specialists.[130] Among the subjects they chose to illumine are catalogues of Arabic names learned in Nablus (Shechem) and its vicinity, and lists of names of Jews of Damascus. Other subjects published later concerned the traditional customs of the *fellahin* under the regime of the *sheikhs*, military service, the fighting force, and the wars between the Kais, tribes originating from northern Arabia, and the Yaman, a loose federation of Bedouin tribes of south Arabian origin, whose conflict dates back to the Muslim conquest of Palestine in 634-638. They also reviewed the subject of traditional clothes and dress, women's local customs, traditional food and beverages, work, marriage, birth, hospitality, family purity, blood disputes, pilgrimage, and annual *ziara* celebrations (festive religious gatherings at holy places and sacred graves, celebrated by Muslims as well as Jews in Arab countries).[131] Other segments of this series of articles described local rulers in Palestine from the sixteenth to the nineteenth century such as Daher al-Umar (1689-1775), a local Bedouin chief and ruler of northern Palestine from 1730 to 1775, and Ibrahim Pasha, the son of the Muhammed Ali (1789-1848), ruler of Egypt who ruled Palestine from 1831 to 1840 as well. A chronological table was appended to the final article to make this period clear for the European reader.[132]

Masterman did not neglect the flora; in one essay he reviews the trees and the bushes of the Holy Land,[133] and describes new plants such as the eucalyptus tree and certain fruit trees, and he attempts to identify biblical trees and bushes. Regarding the sycamore he writes:

> The 'sycamore' of Luke xvii, 6 and 1 Kings x, 27, was not the mulberry nor the maple-sycamore of Europe but the sycamore-fig, a splendid tree rather like a large fig but developing poor fruit, which is found in many parts of the land to-day'. As for the white broom, 'The 'juniper tree' under which Elijah lay (1 Kings xix, 5) in the wilderness, was certainly the familiar ratam, a kind of broom well known in the Jordan valley; it is even to-day burnt by the natives to produce charcoal (Ps., cii, 4)'; and the hyssop: 'What was the 'hyssop' of Ex, xii, 22, 1 Kings iv, 33, John, xix, 29, has been a subject of endless debate'.

This expertise might have been the reason Masterman was asked to write the entry on the grape vine for one of the more important encyclopedias of the Bible.[134]

Archaeology and historical geography

Masterman's enviable skill as a horseman opened to him the remotest recesses of the country, at a time when vehicular traffic was limited to a few main roads: and he traversed the country from end to end and from side to side many a time, learning it 'like a map'; nothing could escape his observant eye.[135] He visited almost every corner of the Holy Land. His curiosity led him to explore and research archaeological sites, and to find and identify biblical sites in Palestine as well as east of the Jordan River.[136] In one article he reports exploring an ancient aqueduct from the Virgin Fountain discovered by the renowned German scholar Conrad Schick. The excavations were actually done by local workers from the Siloam village. Masterman reports on and describes various aqueducts and tunnels and cites the views of other scholars regarding these findings.[137] He also published an article about the aqueduct found at Wadi Qumran and attached two pictures to this particular report.[138]

Masterman penned a scholarly report regarding the site of 'Capernaum' on the northern shores of the Sea of Galilee. This piece reveals his wide-ranging knowledge and expertise, evident from his summary of previous visits and identifications of the site, from the time of Byzantine scholars such as Theodorus (sixth century) through medieval pilgrims and scholars such as Arculfus (seventh century), Willibert (eighth century), Epiphanios (tenth century), Burchard (thirteenth century) and Father Noe (sixteenth century). Citations from the New Testament and Josephus and a detailed description of the site and its names, are found in this article as well.[139] The identification of the biblical *tel* 'Chephirah of Benjamin' (the ruins of a biblical city first mentioned in Joshua ix, 17 as one of the four cities of the Gibeonites) was given serious treatment by Masterman who used it as a tool of historical geography.[140]

One of Masterman's journeys in the northern parts of the Holy Land, accompanied by Macalister, was published as a detailed travelogue. This diary includes scholarly remarks and descriptions of Nablus (Shechem), Beisan (Beit-Shean), Tiberias, the Sea of Galilee, Safed mountain, and the city of Safed. Archaeological sites and discussions on the identity of various sites are presented in this article.[141] Visits and tours to castles and fortifications built during the Jewish revolt against the Romans (67-73 AD) are reported in another paper. It includes a detailed description of the ruins of well fortified and hidden Jewish fortresses where the Galilean rebels held out against the Romans in 66 AD. These are Gabara and Taricheae, situated on a cliff near Safed and Tiberias. Masterman describes each site in detail, with its name, Josephus' account, and a discussion of its identification.[142] A tour in the Judean desert is fully reported in an article entitled 'Notes of a Visit to Engedy, Masada and Jebal Usdum'.[143] On this visit Masterman was accompanied by Prof. Francis Brown (1849-1916) of the American School of Archeology and his students. The journey took place in January 1908, and the report contains times, temperatures, pictures, reports of views, findings, archaeological sites, Bedouin customs, tribal boundary signs, and more.[144]

Research work during the stay in Damascus

The year that Masterman spent in Damascus yielded many finds which were reported in several publications. At 1896 he published a Greek inscription on a column in Damascus[145] and another from the city's Grand Mosque.[146] In a different article Masterman presents a general report on the customs he observed in the city.[147] He sets forth in detail modernization processes there as well. In a paper on the new Damascus railway, two lines are reported in detail, with data on length, routes, stations, and more.[148]

In Damascus Masterman continued to be involved with the exploration and research of the Holy Land. An interesting example is found in his article 'In answer to Dr Bailey' regarding the water in Jacob's Well.[149] Here he applies his knowledge of Arabic by citing Arabic proverbs; he describes the traditions of people from all over the Holy Land coming to drink the well's water. He even respectfully criticizes the ideas of Prof. George Adam Smith (1856-1942)[150] the Scottish scholar and author of the well known book *Historical Geography of the Holy Land* (London 1894; and 26 editions since then).[151]

Medical Achievements and Contribution

Along with his practical medical activities and professional life, Masterman always found the time and energy to continue conducting research and lecturing to distinguished audiences. He had begun medical research before his arrival in Palestine. In 1891 he published articles on the spread of gangrene around the mouth[152] and rodent ulcer,[153] which demonstrate well the scientific resources available to the young Masterman.

Masterman continued his research after his arrival in Jerusalem, and in November 1900 he published an article on the city's smallpox epidemic. Before making any comment on the epidemic, Masterman describes the medical condition of Jerusalem, emphasizing the relatively large number of physicians as well as hospital beds, compared with European cities. Then follows a unique description of the negative attitude of the Jerusalem inhabitants to smallpox, the basic sanitation rules, vaccination, and the Western physician. The article ends with practical advice: 'In conclusion, should any of the readers of this have friends going East this season, I would strongly advise them to insist on re-vaccination for all'.[154]

Early in 1903, Masterman wrote a report on a cholera epidemic that had stricken Palestine in the autumn of the previous year. The article is highly critical of the Turkish authorities. Regarding their unstable quarantine policy: 'It is a system for which there is no redress, and many foreign residents firmly believe it is kept up because, although it half ruins the country as a whole, it brings big fees into the pockets of certain officials'. Still, the inhabitants evaded quarantine in various ways:

> The irony of the situation, moreover, is that all last summer, while the mails, merchandise, and respectable travellers (often coming as direct as possible from England, France, or Germany) were all being delayed and upset by these irritating regulations for admittance at the front door, all the riffraff of the country were passing happily through the back door from infected Egypt. This 'back door' is the overland route.

Meanwhile, the Cholera epidemic and the range of mortality spread:

> On their return to Jerusalem that district was declared infected. Several weeks had meanwhile been lost, and scared fugitives from the town had scattered themselves widely around carrying infection to Jaffa, Lydd, Helom, and numerous villages. What was the actual mortality in Gaza it is impossible to say… there is no possibility of knowing the truth; truth, too, on such a subject is a disagreeable thing to the official's mind, and is usually very deep 'in the well'.

Different cases were reported to drive home, by means of anecdotal evidence, the dilemmas that Western physicians faced. Masterman notes several traditional medications, and a strange anecdote on rumours of killing patients as a way to stop the epidemic.[155]

Tropical diseases, parasitology, fevers and malaria

During his long period of practicing medicine in Palestine, Masterman specialized in treating tropical diseases. He shared his knowledge and experience by writing articles for professional journals such as *The Journal of Hygiene*. Masterman reviewed the medical conditions of Jerusalem as a city that attracted thousands of visitors and pilgrims yearly. The diseases and maladies that struck the city's visitors and inhabitants, such as Palestinian malaria and dengue fever which spread in 1912, are described as well.[156] In 1913, in another article, he describes in detail typhus fever, Jericho boil, ulcerative stomatitis and enteric fever.[157] Some years before, in 1908, Masterman had reported on human parasites in Palestine, thereby revealing yet another direction of his medical expertise: parasitology.[158]

In a short article published in 1906, Masterman reviewed haemoglobinuric fever and informed readers of several cases in Palestine. The article opening tells about its importance:

> It is, I think, not known that haemoglobinuric, or 'black fever', often occurs in Palestine. Not only is the place not mentioned in the accounts I have seen of the geographical distribution of this disease, but in Allbutt's System of Medicine it is stated, 'in Asia the disease is practically unknown'.[159]

Other fevers were very common in Palestine in the nineteenth century and were described by other physicians, mainly Dr Thomas Chaplin, the former director of the English Mission Hospital in Jerusalem.[160] Chaplin spent much time treating patients and researching the disease. He published extensively on this subject in an article published serially.[161] This article is regarded by some scholars as the first scientific paper sent from Palestine, and it reflects the acute form of the disease in nineteenth-century Palestine.[162] However, the majority of fevers in Palestine in general, and Jerusalem in particular, were identified as malaria by most European physicians visiting or practicing in Palestine.[163]

Malaria, which was well established in Palestine, captured Masterman's attention and in 1905 he reported on the existence of the disease and of the Anopheles mosquito in the country.[164] Other foreign physicians,[165] and local colleagues such as Wheeler, reported on malaria as well.[166] Masterman's efforts and research into malaria, mainly in 1912-1913, appear sophisticated and modern, and eventually became very important for his research as well as for the studies of other scholars. Masterman took blood specimens from hundreds of his Jewish patients with fever cases at his hospital and dispensaries to be tested for the malaria parasites.[167] He praises his fellow physicians, gives credit to other colleagues and researchers such as Peter Muelens (b. 1874)[168] and John Cropper (1864-1916),[169] and describes his research in minute detail. On account of his expertise and personal interest, Masterman paid special attention to malaria, the presence of the Anopheles mosquito, and the draining of the swamps, as well as the seasonal water system, in an article for the annual report of the Ministry of Health for 1921.[170]

Other diverse medical activities and posts

In August 1904 Masterman gave a lecture titled 'Jerusalem from the sanitary point of view', which was partly published in *Home Words for Jerusalem*, a publication of the London Jews Society.[171] Another article is 'History of the Jerusalem medicinal mission', in which Masterman reviews the work and the contribution of the British Missionary medical team.[172] This article is one of several reports published in the Society's journal on the work of the mission hospital.[173]

Masterman's rich practical experience and medical knowledge, and his acquaintance with the work of his predecessors, mainly Dr Thomas Chaplin,[174] were presented to the scientific community in a series of articles published in the *Palestine Exploration Fund Quarterly Statement*[175]and later compiled in a booklet named *Hygiene and Disease in Palestine in Modern and in Biblical Times.*[176] Even after he left Palestine, because of the outbreak of the First World War, Masterman continued to report on and interpret the country's medical conditions. This is evident in his review[177] of the first annual report of the British Mandate medical services in Palestine, tracing the transformation of the Ottoman public health system into its British form. Other issues in the report such as diseases, demographic statistics (birth and death rates), hospitals and their geographical distribution, research institutions, nursing services, and school public health services are described in detail.

During the years he spent in England, more especially from 1920, Masterman was an active member of the British Medical Association (BMA), the professional association of physicians in the United Kingdom founded by Sir Charles Hastings (1810-1888), which represents doctors from all branches of medicine.[178] In 1934-5 he held the position of Joint Honorary Secretary of the Metropolitan Counties Branch of the BMA.

Masterman's investigations, reflected in his many publications, attest that he was a vigorous researcher and talented writer. A review of his work shows his contribution to Jerusalem studies, and his knowledge of the history of the Holy Land, archaeology, social anthropology, the contemporaneous development of Jerusalem and settlement of Jews in the Holy Land, demography, political science (internal and international), hydrology, Dead Sea and Judean desert sciences, Galilee studies, botany, and epigraphy.

We have chosen to focus on three aspects of his work:

Medicine - Masterman's contribution to the understanding of malaria was profound. Alone among his contemporaries, Masterman has been praised and his work studied in detail by a present-day expert in epidemiology and preventive medicine.

'The result of the extra one year blood survey in Jerusalem, allows an examination of the seasonal trend of the Malaria in Jerusalem and the frequency and relative proportions of the different species of malaria parasite'.[179]

Holy Land research - Masterman is well known among archaeologists, climatologists, geographers, historians of medicine, and historians of other aspects of the Holy Land.[180] His measurement of the level of the Dead Sea[181] and especially his conclusive publication[182] are important for scholars, hydrologists, and geographers. The data collected then remains essential for research to the present day.[183] His booklet: *Hygiene and Disease in Palestine in Modern and in Biblical Times*[184] is one of the most important sources for scholars examining the history of medicine in early modern Palestine.[185]

Masterman's contemporary, Sir George Adam Smith, evaluated Masterman's work in a preface he wrote to Masterman's book *Studies in Galilee* in 1909: 'Altogether, Dr. Masterman has laboured for sixteen or seventeen years [and later nine more years, from 1934 to 1943] in the East. His numerous papers in journals devoted to the history or geography of the Holy Land prove his acquaintance with the literature, ancient and modern, and have been largely used by experts. Very few know the recent history of the land or the life of the people like himself'.[186]

Politics – Masterman's understanding of internal politics in Palestine and international relations was unique and helped the mission to develop projects, to improve medical services in Safed, Damascus, and Jerusalem, and to enhance the influence of the mission and of the community of Britons in the Holy Land.

Dr Walter Henry Anderson (1869-1937)

'I feel I am not a man of the words. I have not been accustomed to speaking, so, I am sure, you will bear with me if I try…'.[187] These were the words of the British physician, Dr Walter Henry Anderson, in a public address he made in London, in which he was asked to describe his remarkable achievements as a Medical Doctor among the Jewish People of Palestine.

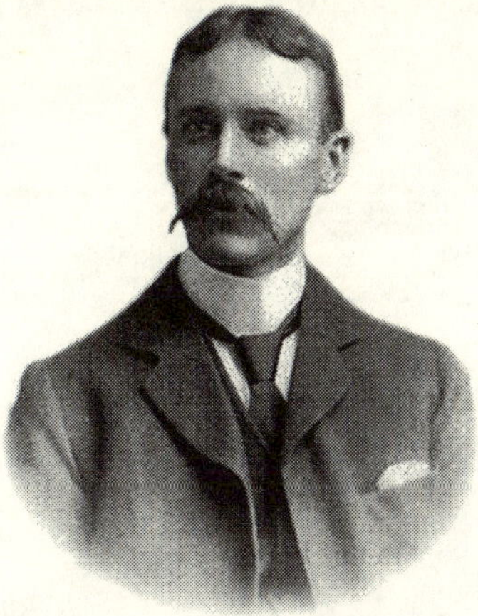

Figure 17 - Dr Walter Henry Anderson

Anderson was born in 1869 in Burton upon Trent and at the age of 24 he joined the ranks of the London Jews Society. That same year, he was appointed Medical Missionary and was sent to Palestine, arriving in Jerusalem on January 18, 1894. Following three months in Jerusalem, he took up his duties at the Society's mission station in Safed on April 6.[188] Anderson set to work with enormous energy, declaring that he saw his position in Safed as his life's vocation. His first recommendation was to open a small hospital of six beds immediately, and at the same time to continue the efforts to establish the large hospital then being proposed. The London Jews Society approved his recommendation and at the end of 1895 he rented a building to be used as a hospital for a period of three years; it opened in February 1896.[189]

Soon enough, the modest medical institution became too cramped for its many patients. By 1895 a suitable compound was located close by the Jewish quarter in Safed, and in the summer of 1900 the General Committee of the London Jews Society authorized the immediate establishment of the Out patients' Department of the still-to-be-built Hospital.[190] On May 31, 1904, the new hospital was inaugurated. It soon acquired a place of honour in the city and was crowded with Jewish patients. During the summer of 1905 the number of patients applying for medical care reached a peak of 302 (out of about 6,000 Jewish inhabitants) in one day.

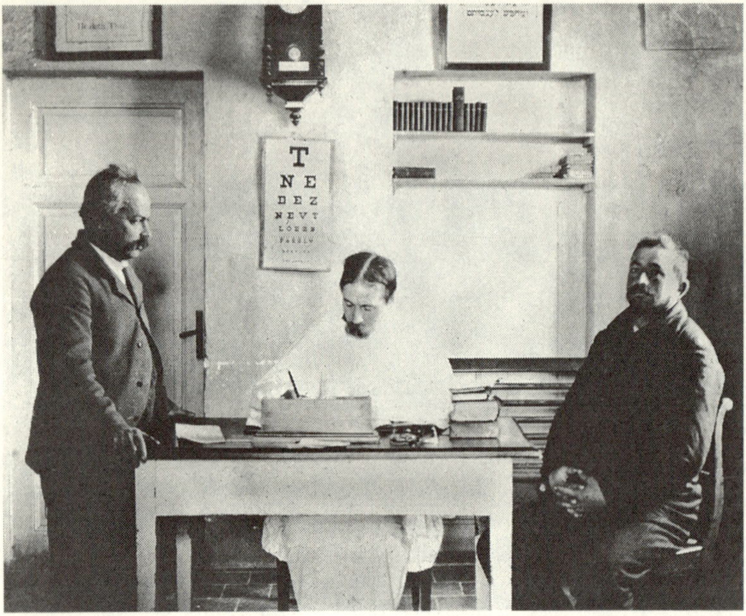

Figure 18 - Anderson in his consulting room in 1906

In 1895, Anderson married a Miss Robertson. She suffered from poor health, and four years after they married and after a stay at the northern town of Haifa in the hope that the change might benefit her health, Mrs. Anderson died. She was laid to rest in the little German cemetery in Haifa, and Anderson was left with two infant children, Four years later Anderson remarried.[191]

Anderson was often in a quandary about his role as a physician alongside his duties as a missionary. He wrote several times to the Society's journal concerning his doubts, describing the temptations that he had to face. He worried about thinking too much about the philanthropic side of the work. While he thought it would be marvellous to be able to relieve suffering, it would be deplorable if that were all that people like him thought of: 'My friends, I can tell you that there is a real temptation to think too much, perhaps, of this side. Will you, therefore, pray that we medical missionaries may be not only medical officers, but real medical missionaries'?[192] During fund-raising tours for the hospital in England, Anderson shared with his audience his rich acquaintance with the Jews of Safed. A useful means was to report changes of heart towards Christianity in some Jewish individuals. In 1899 he wrote:

> …Here I hold in my hand what is called Cherem – a ban of excommunication, published at the instigation of a prominent Safed Jew… When I first went there we were met with great opposition from the Jews, especially from the leaders of the people; and this Jew that I refer to, was one of the chief of our opponents. Two or three years after the publication of this Cherem, I met him… and we spoke together for… an hour or two. Eighteen months later I again met this Jew [who wrote me as follows:] I am fully convinced of the truth of Christianity. If I am a Jew by flesh, I am, I feel, a Christian in heart….[193]

With the outbreak of the First World War Anderson was obliged to leave his post in Safed. In 1915, he joined the Royal Army Medical Corps (R.A.M.C), in which he served until the end of the war.[194] In January 1920, he returned to Palestine to resume his work at the hospital in Safed. Soon after, in the autumn of that year, he was compelled to return to England on health grounds. A year later the London Jews Society felt it wise to transfer the work in Safed to the Scottish mission already established there. Anderson did some services for the Society in England and for a short time in New Zealand. But his health forced him to reduce his work load. He retired to live at Worthing, where he died in 1937.[195]

Discussion

From the establishment of the London Jews Society's medical institutions until the outbreak of the First World War, the physicians' scholarly activities, initiatives and research included the following:

The early British physicians in Jerusalem from the 1830s were occupied in erecting the dispensary and hospital in the city; establishing connections with the local Ottoman regime; gaining the trust of the members of the Jewish community; and struggling against the rabbis' proscriptions. These tasks took up all their spare time, as they dedicated their hours to treating fellow emissaries, combating their own diseases, and working as devoted missionaries. In the 1840s and 1850s, Dr Edward Macgowan, founder of the English Mission Hospital and its first director (1842-1860), performed the budding research, including medical studies such as descriptions of the most prevalent diseases and of the city's sanitary conditions. He also found the energy to make tours for a few surveys and to monitor the climate as well. The physicians performing under Macgowan until 1860 were mostly devoted employees with no time to spare for other activities. Some reported to the Society's committee in London, and their reports were frequently published in the Society's journal, but they could not manage anything more.

Chaplin represents the second category of activities. By the time he took up his post in Jerusalem, the hospital was well established. The medical staff were well organized and functioned very smoothly; the health of the members of the mission was better, and the local Ottoman authorities in some way supported the hospital's activities. The dispute with the rabbis of Jerusalem was more moderate. At the end of that decade, the Palestine Exploration Fund began operations in Palestine. Consequently, and in keeping with Chaplin's character, inquisitiveness and energy, he managed to gain some expertise in medical research in a variety of topics such as common fevers and leprosy. His colleagues in the PEF encouraged him to make use of his many skills and to take tours for medical and research purposes. Scholars in various fields were swept up by his enthusiasm, and shared with him their knowledge and also their scientific equipment. In this way, he obtained a climate measurement kit, which enabled him to make an accurate evaluation of the climate in Jerusalem for 25 years. His archaeologist associates changed him from an amateur to a professional archaeologist. His broad knowledge of Bible, linguistics, history, and geography were fully utilized for fund-raising and establishing medical institutions in addition to those built by the mission.

Wheeler epitomizes the third category: a man of hard work who dedicated himself to the establishment of the new hospital. Indeed, the Society's committee in London presumably appointed him as a physician, a missionary, and a technocrat, rather than a scholar like Chaplin. Consequently, and in accordance with his nature and abilities, Wheeler's research and writing were not remarkable.

Masterman worked under Wheeler for 18 years before becoming the hospital's director. He did not have overall responsibility, and the possibility exists that he might have been frustrated, having as his superior a less talented scholar, and a man with less charisma. Nevertheless, Masterman used his spare time in a variety of research activities, and continued the scholarly heritage of his predecessor, Dr Thomas Chaplin. Masterman specialized in the research of malaria, made archaeological excavations, was an expert philologist, and made many research tours, publishing his findings and conclusions in numerous books and papers.

After the conclusion of the First Word War and establishment of the British Mandate over Palestine, there was no longer a need for the London Jews Society's scholars, as the British Government dispatched its own district physicians to furnish medical reports, and scholars could travel freely throughout the country, conducting their research. Accordingly, after the war, the physicians of the London Jews Society's medical institution devoted their energies to medical treatment only.

IMPACT

Other Hospitals built in Late Ottoman Palestine

As a result of the pioneering medical enterprise of the London Jews Society, the competition among the Great Powers over holdings in the Holy Land found expression in the sphere of medicine as well. Gradually, Jewish medical institutions were established so that Jews would not become patients in Christian institutions. At the same time, European institutions began to set up additional modern hospitals, in part to establish a national presence in the face of the efficient British hospitals. On the eve of the First World War, there were more than two dozen hospitals functioning in Palestine, and Jerusalem itself had some fifteen modern medical institutions. This chapter reviews the history of the main hospitals that were erected during the nineteenth century and up until the First World War. The changes that occurred in the process of modernization in the Land of Israel are examined and the valuable contributions made by the medical institutions of the London Jews Society are discussed.

Protestant Medical Activity, Institutions and Politics

The Anglo-Prussian Bishopric

The formal activities of the Protestant world in Palestine commenced with the early attempts of the emissaries of the London Jews Society to get a hold in Jerusalem, mainly with the founding of the mission post in the city by John Nicolayson in the autumn of 1833. But a joint Bishopric for the English and Prussians, which was established in 1841, laid the basis for Protestant activity in Palestine during the nineteenth century. The legal status of Protestants in the Ottoman Empire improved. Health, education, charity and welfare institutions were established, attracting thousands of travellers, pilgrims, scholars and scientists to Palestine.

The initiator of the Anglo-Prussian Bishopric was Christian Karl Josias von Bunsen (1791-1860), a friend and confidant of Friedrich Wilhelm IV, King of Prussia (1796-1861). [1] Bunsen, a native of Waldeck in the Kingdom of Hessen, who served in the Prussian Foreign Office at the Papal Court, was forced to leave his position in Rome on the order of the Pope due to his involvement in a quarrel between Protestant Prussia and the Vatican. This incident spurred Bunsen to attempt to undermine the power of the Catholic Church, which he regarded as the source of his misfortune, by strengthening the status of the Protestant Church. The connection between Bunsen's frustration and his plans to establish a Protestant Bishopric in Jerusalem seems quite obvious.

Friedrich Wilhelm saw in the relationship between the English government and the Church a model for imitation, and therefore responded with enthusiasm to Bunsen's proposals to institutionalize the cooperation between Protestant Anglicans and their German brethren. Bunsen was sent to London and soon gained Queen Victoria's (1819-1901) approval for his plan. The parties negotiated mutually agreeable formula regarding the division of authority within the future Bishopric, and decided that the Bishop of Jerusalem would be appointed alternately. The Archbishop of Canterbury, the head of the Anglican Church, had the right to veto any candidate proposed by the Prussian crown.[2] According to the proposal of the King of Prussia, the British were the first to put forward their candidate, and they selected Michael Solomon Alexander (1799-1845), a converted Jew and veteran missionary of the London Jews Society.[3]

On January 21, 1842 Bishop Alexander entered Jerusalem, with clear instructions to devote direct efforts 'to the conversion of the Jews, to their protection, and to their useful employment'.[4] The arrival of the Bishop, the heart and soul of the London Jews Society, raised great hopes in the hearts of its members. The Society lost no time taking advantage of the credit reaped jointly with the Anglo-Prussian Bishopric in Jerusalem, to further its aims.

Soon they built the first hospital in the Holy Land, the first western educational institutes in the country, and completed the building of the first Protestant church in the Turkish Empire. But the era of Bishop Alexander in the Holy Land ended on November 23, 1845 when he passed away while en-route to visit the Jewish communities in Egypt.

After Bishop Alexander's death, it was the King of Prussia's turn to select his candidate for heading the Protestant Bishopric in Jerusalem. Friedrich Wilhelm accepted Bunsen's proposal, who by then was the Prussian Ambassador in London, and offered the position to Samuel Gobat, a missionary who was then serving in the ranks of the Church Missionary Society. Gobat, a native of the village of Cremines in the Jura Mountains of the Bern canton in Switzerland, had received his training at the Mission in Basle. At the time the position was offered to him, he was serving in Malta, with years of activity as missionary in the Near East and especially in Ethiopia to his credit. Gobat willingly accepted the appointment, entering the gates of Jerusalem at the end of December 1846.[5]

Gobat was sometimes suspected of having no particular affection for Jews, especially in view of the hurdles he put in the way of those wishing to convert to Christianity. It is recorded in his biography that deep in his heart he dearly loved the Jews of Jerusalem, but because of his knowledge of human nature, he chose not to exhibit his true feelings and to refrain from emotionalism. In his own words: 'I tremble whenever the missionaries send me a convert [Jew], for either he is insincere from the beginning, or, if he commences by being honest and in earnest, he will soon be spoilt by the flattery of the friends of Israel in England.'.[6] At the beginning of 1847 he wrote in his diary, that to the best of his knowledge, his superiors had not sent him to work only among the Jews. He felt it was his duty to be a debtor also to 'the wise and to the ignorant, Greeks [Orthodox], Romanists [Catholics], Armenians, Turks [Muslims], &c'.[7]

Apart from his direct activities within the local Arab population, the Bishop encouraged, and at times even initiated, the arrival of additional Protestant parties which he intended for work among various communities in the country. One such institution maintaining a presence in Palestine was the 'Deaconesses of Kaiserswerth'.

Deaconesses of Kaiserswerth's Hospital

The founder of the Institute of the Deaconesses of Kaiserswerth was the German Pastor Theodor Fliedner (1800-1864).[8] At the early age of 22, Fliedner became the Parson of the Protestant Parish of Kaiserswerth (today in the German city of Düsseldorf) and was engaged in community work. He was the founder of the first German prison society and helped female ex-prisoners to find their way back to society. He was a pioneer in favour of professions for women and founded an institution in which women were trained to serve as social workers, educators and nurses. He gained sponsors, recruited candidates and launched the Diakonissen-Mutterhaus, a training centre for women, in his congregation in Kaiserswerth in 1838.[9]

Fliedner had in mind to transform nursing from an originally male profession to a truly feminine one in his institution for training nurses in Kaiserswerth. A profound understanding of the special character of women and empathy for the needs of sick people provided the foundation for the ethics of the nursing profession well beyond the range of the Deaconesses idea. A particularly valuable witness of this activity was Florence Nightingale (1820-1910), the founder of modern nursing in England who spent several months of training in Kaiserswerth.[10]

In 1851, when a typhoid fever epidemic spread in Palestine, also finding victims among its Anglican-Protestant community, Bishop Gobat turned to Fliedner to send two graduate of his institute to help with the medical work in Jerusalem. After getting the blessings of his friend, Friedrich Wilhelm IV, King of Prussia, Fliedner contacted the London Jews Society and proposed to send a delegation of four sisters to help the medical institution of the Society as well. In April 1851, after the London Jews Society had accepted his proposal and even paid traveling expenses, Fliedner himself accompanied the foursome to Jerusalem. With extraordinary fundraising efforts, the institute in Kaiserswerth managed to establish and run many educational and medical institutions in Palestine.

The modest Deaconesses hospital within the walls of Jerusalem was opened by Fliedner on May 2, 1851, in a small building acquired for Fliedner by the King of Prussia. The sisters who devoted themselves to the education of Arab girls established a small school on the same compound.[11]

The sisters brought with them a wide ranging stock of medicines. And, since one of them was a schooled apothecary trained in preparing prescriptions, the number of patients grew constantly and exceeded the original capacity of eight to ten bedridden patients. Dr Macgowan, the founder of the British mission hospital, was called in to administer the medical treatment. But the major obstacle for the sisters was conversing with the patients, who often spoke only Arabic, Amharic, Russian, Greek, Hebrew or Yiddish, all unknown languages for the Deaconesses. Therefore, they received some organized Arabic lessons once a week.

On January 27, 1868 the Deaconesses inaugurated their new school building of Talitha Kumi. The former school rooms in the Jerusalem's old city compound were converted for the use of the hospital. About 40 bedridden patients were treated daily and more than 500 sick people could get assistance during the year. Dr Thomas Chaplin, the second director of the British mission hospital, who replaced Macgowan in 1860, was forced to leave his unpaid post due to his own health. The sisters turned to Dr Max Sandreczki (1839-1899) who already had a great reputation in Jerusalem.[12] However, his salary was a heavy burden for the finances of the institute and in due course he was replaced by the German Templar physician Dr Samuel Hoffmann (1849-1903).

In the mid 1880s, the hospital began to deteriorate and to suffer from diminished attendance due to lack of funds. The sisters started to charge a fee for their treatment, and this eased the situation in some ways, but much more was needed. The lack of a proper operating theatre made advanced surgical work impossible. Moreover, the primitive sanitary installations in the old hospital itself and in the immediate vicinity caused avoidable infections. The building, erected in 1851, had been the only location available at the time. Since then, however, house building was increasing outside the city walls and the security situation there had much improved. Therefore, the Deaconesses decided to establish a new hospital outside the walls. A property not far from the Talitha Kumi School was located, and financial contributions were collected in Europe.[13]

The plans for the new hospital of the Deaconesses in Jerusalem were undertaken by the Berlin architects Schwartzkopff and Theissing. In 1890, they purchased the plot and the building was begun with the foundation, the cellar rooms and a large cistern. Architect Theodor Sandel (1845-1902), a German resident of the German Templar colony in Jerusalem, was in charge of its construction.

The new hospital was opened with a great dedication party on July 3, 1892. The structure consisted of three buildings: one wing faced north and was two stories high; the second wing faced west and had three floors, since it stood on lower ground; the entrance was in the third wing which connected the two others at a sharp angle. The entire complex was of equal height, its middle part emphasized by an arcade at ground floor and a pointed bell tower which rose above a gable, decorated with a dove, the symbol of the order. The building was planned to accommodate 90 bedridden patients, in addition to housing the clinics, pharmacy, and offices. The building still stands today, on the corner of Ha'Neviim and Strauss St. in the heart of Jerusalem.[14] The old building inside the walls is owned by the Maronites and serves as their community centre.

Jesus-Hilfe Leper's Hospital

Leprosy was a common disease in the East, and Jerusalem was home to many lepers during the nineteenth century. They lived in horrible conditions in their separate huts near the Zion Gate and were not provided with any medical treatment at all. This situation was well described by a few European travellers and visitors such as Titus Tobler. He described the symptoms and progress of the disease by writing: 'I saw men without beards... People without teeth... and patients without fingers... the urine is yellow and the excrement is black'. He reported that the strongest married and had healthy babies. Death from this terrible disease was sudden. The causes of the disease were unknown at the time, but Tobler assumed that it was of a genetic condition (an early and unique remark for the mid-nineteenth century). Although there was no cure, he listed some treatments: bloodletting, leeches, purgatives, bath, fast, magic, and use of substances such as mercury and snakes.[15]

Tobler, in a somewhat ironic remark concluded this unpleasant subject on a humanitarian note. How is it, he wondered, that 'the British, who show overdone sympathy towards the Jews, are apathetic to this disaster... A human, compassionate heart would have found the way to get them back to human society. Humanity has many means to fight leprosy'.[16] Indeed, in 1875, Dr Gerhard Hansen published his discovery of the bacteria which generates the disease that was later named after him.[17]

Nearly half a century after Tobler's note, Dr Thomas Chaplin described leprosy in his book 'On Some Diseases Mentioned in the Bible':

> Of all the diseases which afflict humanity, leprosy is one of the most terrible. It infects the whole body, producing hideous distortion of the features, falling of the hair of the eyebrows and face, swellings, ulcerations, contractions of the fingers and toes, which often drop off, leaving only the stumps of the hands or feet, loss of sensation, so that the affected parts can be burned without the patient feeling it, diminution of muscular power, hoarseness of voice, the sufferer speaking in a strange, unearthly whisper, a repulsive odour, and lingering death, which is usually preceded by a kind of dysentery.[18]

He added a learned discussion in which he cited all the biblical citations relating to the 'tzara'ath' (leprosy) and other skin diseases. The discussion included arguments in Greek, Latin, Hebrew, and Arabic relating to ancient and modern medical descriptions. On the identification of the disease and the relation with other skin diseases he wrote that

> From ancient times down to a quite recent period, persons suffering from other loathsome diseases beside true 'leprosy' or elephantiasis were banished from their homes and sent to live amongst the leper. It is said that in Europe, at one time, as many as 75 per cent of the inmates of the Lazar house were not afflicted with elephantiasis.[19]

Twenty years after Chaplin, Dr Ernst Masterman claimed that Leprosy was not a common disease but that it infected all classes – Muslims, Jews and Christians: 'All over Palestine there are not more than 250 lepers, most of them segregated in Jerusalem'.[20] He affirmed Chaplin's identification of the disease and mentioned that in biblical times leprosy was the name for a wide range of skin diseases then considered contagious. With the passage of time and changing conditions, the illness called 'leprosy' in the nineteenth century was not necessarily the same disease mentioned in the Bible.

The initiators of the first modern Lepers hospital in Jerusalem were Baroness Augusta Keffenbrinck-Ascheraden and her husband Baron Wilhelm Friedrich of East Prussia. During a tour they took in 1865 guided by Dr Thomas Chaplin, the couple wished to ease the distress of the lepers by establishing a sanatorium for them in Jerusalem. After returning back home, the Baroness raised the necessary funds for the project and contacted Samuel Gobat, the Protestant Bishop in Jerusalem. She asked him to head the medical institution and to form a committee of prominent Protestant figures in Jerusalem. One of its members, Georg Rosen (1820-1891) the Prussian Consul in Jerusalem, bought a plot of land out side the city walls by the new Jewish neighborhood 'Machane Israel' (today 20 Agron St.). The plans for the construction were prepared by the well known Jerusalem architect Conrad Schick.[21]

On May 20, 1867, a Leper hospital in Jerusalem was inaugurated with Dr Chaplin as the chief physician. The Moravian Church in Herrnhut, that took part in establishing the hospital, nominated as the administrator its emissary Freidrich Wilhelm Conrad Theodor Tappe (1824-1897). The two storey building accommodated 12 lepers. It was filled with mainly Muslims, only after the Turkish governor expelled the lepers from their huts in the old city.[22] From the reports and descriptions of the patients, and the treatment provided, along with the fact that Chaplin was consulting outside experts, several researchers have concluded that the treatment in the hospital would be relevant even now.[23] In the yearly report of 1876, Chaplin reported that in the hospital's first decade, 50 patients were hospitalized, 36 of them males and 14 females. Of those 50 patients, 12 died, 20 left the hospital and 18 were still on the premises.[24]

In 1881 the management of the hospital was transferred to the Moravian Church. In 1882 its committee decided to establish a new hospital according to Chaplin's recommendation. The main reasons were its proximity to the city and the space needed for Chaplin's medical objectives. The piece of land chosen for the new hospital was the one already bought by Tappe in 1874. It was half an hour walking distance from the old site and near the German Templar colony of Rephaim (17 Marcus St. of today).[25] These plans too, were drawn up by Conrad Schick. In 1884 the work began.

The cornerstone was laid on May 9, 1885 and the inauguration of the hospital took place on April 24, 1887. Above the front entrance engraved in stone was the Hospital's name 'Jesus Hilfe' (Jesus Help). The large modern building was built on 12 acres of land. Some of the needs of the hospital were supplied by the vegetables and fruits that were cultivated in its garden, as well as by the large herd of livestock. In 1905 the hospital reached its full capacity of 60 patients.[26]

On January 1, 1886, Dr Chaplin left his position as head of the English Mission Hospital and the Leper's Hospital in Jerusalem after 20 years of service and returned to London. His successor in the leper hospital was Dr Adalbert Einsler (1848-1919) a specialist in eye diseases, of Hungarian origin, who practised in several Jewish and German hospitals in Jerusalem starting in 1881.

The Marienstift Kinderhospital

History of the concept of children's hospitals

The fact that sick children were sent to adult hospitals in European countries even from the time of the Renaissance was repeatedly denounced as 'a scandal and disgrace'. In some cases it was recorded that up to eight children were forced to share one bed, with over 90 percent dying as a result of infection.[27] The first known outpatient dispensary for sick children was established in 1769 by George Armstrong (1719-1789) in London, and was forced to close in 1872 for lack of public interest and support.[28] The importance of the dispensary lay in its new concept that sick children require a special type of medical institution, distinct from those of adults, to administer advice and medicines gratis to children of the 'Industrious Poor, from birth to the age 10 or 12 years' and for the aim of saving 'a great many lives very useful to the Public'. The institute treated 35,000 children in 12 years.[29]

In 1816, the Royal Infirmary for Children was established in London containing three departments focusing on outpatients. The *Kinderkrankeninstitut* (Institution for Sick Children) was established as a philanthropic institution in Vienna in 1788. A similar Institution was founded in Germany in 1837. According to some scholars the first children's hospital in the world 'Hôpital des Enfants Malades', was established in Paris in 1802 when the orphanage 'Maison de l'Enfant Jésus' was transform into a children's hospital.[30]

Guidelines for the ideal children's hospital were laid down by Carl Rauchfuss (1835-1915), a German-Russian pediatrician: 'If one were simply to build children's hospitals along exactly the same construction and with the same furnishing, equipment and organization as the general hospitals, then it would not be worthwhile building them at all'. Rauchfuss added that the main idea is to unite all elements of child care under one roof, and the ideal is a capacity of ten beds and 500 hundred outpatients per 10,000 inhabitants. There should be certain structural elements in such a hospital: a separate outpatient department with a different physician from that in the inpatient departments; observation or quarantine ward and isolation houses serving every conceivable form of diseases, including mixed cases; play and gymnastic halls for physiotherapy; and garden areas.[31]

The Hospital in Jerusalem

The prominent figure behind the children's hospital in Jerusalem was Dr Max Sandreczki. His father, Carl Sandreczki (1810-1892), a missionary of the British 'Church Missionary Society' came to Palestine with 12 year old Max in 1851. In the following years, Max Sandreczki left to study medicine in Munich, Tübingen and Würzburg and after graduation, worked in a well known Kinderpoliklinik in Munich. In 1866 he joined the Prussian army (fighting the Austrians at that time) and served as medical director of a field hospital. One year later, he left with his wife for the Holy

Land and was appointed director of the Hospital of the German Deaconesses of Kaiserswerth in Jerusalem.[32] (see above).

The idea of funding a children's hospital in Jerusalem was brought up for the first time in 1869[33] during a visit by the Crown Prince Friedrich Wilhelm of Prussia (1831-1888 in days to come the German Kaiser Friedrich III), which was guided by Carl Sandreczki. However, this idea did not come to fruition for another 3 years. In 1871, the Archduke of Mecklenburg Schwerin (1823-1883) and his wife Princess Marie of Schwarzburg Rudolstadt (1850-1922), arrived in Jerusalem as visitors. The distinguished couple were impressed by Dr Sandreczki and his wife Johanna Alida Hofs and decided to support their dream.[34]

A written proposal for the establishment of a children's hospital was sent to Schwerin in February 1872. According to Sandreczki there were at that time in Jerusalem 6 hospitals (in addition to the Leper hospital, which was considered by Sandreczki as a shelter): German Deaconesses - 40 beds, Russian - 60 beds, Greek Patriarch - 45 beds, Rothschild 20-30 beds, English -30 beds and a small French hospital. In Sandreczki's opinion, all of the hospitals except the German hospital, were motivated by nationalism and religious rules and did not accept children as inpatients. Sandreczki mentioned the moral and health implications of hospitalizing adults and children together. He also discussed the great need and the main medical problems afflicting children in the Holy Land in general and in Jerusalem in particular, e.g children who have leprosy.[35]

The schema of establishing the hospital was presented to the Archduke of Mecklenburg Schwerin and his wife, in February 26, 1872 in Jerusalem. It was approved three days later, by granting 1000 Marks annually, as long as the institution was open (unless the hospital was not established by July 1, 1873, in which case the donation expired).[36]

The hospital, named after the princess, was opened in 1872, in one of the earliest houses to be built outside the city walls (29 Ha'Neviim St. of today). It contained six beds, two cradles and two beds for accompanying mothers. It treated 107 patients in the first year with 2,803 hospital days of operation and these figures increased over the years. The hospital's rules and regulations were very humane e.g. no missionary attempts or conversion of the children or their parents were allowed. The hospital was required to serve children from all ethnic and religious groups. Sandreczki, employed without any payment, supplied the medical treatment to the children who suffered from the various diseases that afflicted the Holy Land, and carried out the surgical operations. Even though these were complex operations, the mortality rate in the hospital was rather low: 5 children out of 107 treated in first year died and 9 out of 548 in 1898. Sandreczki maintained a high quality of medical care, despite the distance from Europe. Sandreczki was considered as an advanced physician and surgeon. His fresh and original ideas, observations and methods were published and attracted much interest in Europe.[37]

The hospital faced severe financial problems over the years, but figures like Otto von Bismarck (1815-1898), the German Chancellor, donated generously to keep the hospital functioning. Kaiser Wilhelm II (1859-1941) was likewise a contributor, having donated 1500 marks. The hospital's financial difficulties were in part due to its policy of not proselytizing. As a result, it was not connected to any major European organization. The budget was balanced in 1890 after Sandreczki attracted wealthy friends and contributors in Europe and the United States. The hope for a significant contribution that would enable the building of a new modern hospital was turned down by Kaiser Wilhelm II after a visit he made with his wife Auguste Victoria (1858-1921) in Jerusalem in 1898. Notwithstanding being decorated by the Kaiser, Sandreczki did not receive the money he needed. After the Kaiser left the city, the ruler of Jerusalem ordered the closure of the hospital, but Sandreczki refused and continue to run the institution. On June 22, 1899, sick and disappointed, Sandreczki committed suicide. The hospital was closed down after several months during which it was run down by his widow, Johanna.[38]

Max Sandreczki was an educated and talented physician. He applied a modern attitude towards the children and mother relationship in paediatric medicine. He spoke 7 languages, and wrote, as early as in 1872, that fungus and bacteria create infectious diseases. He conducted research and published an article on leprosy which was translated into English and was also published in the

Lancet. That he was a paediatric surgeon implies high standards of medical and surgical practice in his hospital, which not only compared favourably with Western European standards, but was in some aspects, even more advanced. According to some scholars his medical institution was an 'implant' of a Western institution into a society that was 'mediaeval in character'.[39]

Order of St. John's Ophthalmic Hospital

Eye diseases and ailments were prevalent in nineteenth century Palestine. The rural population, village communities and nomadic Bedouin suffered from eye inflammations and diseases far more than the urban population. This reflected a combination of the poverty, ignorance, and neglect that characterized the Middle East as a whole at the time. Eye diseases usually broke out with the coming of the spring, and lasted throughout the summer. Trachoma was among the wide spread diseases in Palestine before and during the British Mandate. Eye injuries had a cultural dimension as well, especially these resulting from work accidents, rock-throwing in disputes within traditional herding and village cultures, eye injuries in battle, and even deliberate grievous injury to one's enemies as an accepted 'rule of war'. In November 1886, the first modern eye hospital was inaugurated in the Holy Land, treating hundreds of patients every month. Still, into the early years of the twentieth century most Palestine residents contracted *Ophthalmia* due to poor sanitary and hygienic conditions including crowded housing and the sharing of clothes, bedding, and towels by entire families.[40]

The initiator of the eye hospital was the English branch of the Order of St. John of Jerusalem. The Order, which had been revived in England as a Catholic organization and soon after became an Anglican institution, tried to promote the establishment of a 'Hospice and Ophthalmic Dispensary in Jerusalem'. Various distinguished English gentlemen were involved in this initiative, including Sir Edmund Lechmere (1826-1894), General Secretary of the Order at that time. In December 1876, he published an address, asking that a site in Jerusalem be found for the building of an English hospital. The British representative in Constantinople, requested such ground from the Ottoman government on behalf of the Order, but no such site was available.[41]

In 1881, Noel Temple Moore (1833-1903), the British Consul in Jerusalem, located another site in Jerusalem and Albert Edward Prince of Wales (1841-1910) was asked by the Order to submit his request to Musurus Pasha, the Turkish Ambassador in London. High level politics were involved, as high as the Sultan himself.[42] Eventually a year later, in April 1882, the Sultan granted a firman for the establishment of the Ophthalmic Hospital and Dispensary in Jerusalem, stating as follows:

> To Rauf Pasha[43] my Noble Governor of the Sandjak [province] of Jerusalem, bearer of my Imperial Orders of the Medjidije of the Second Class and of the Osmanieh of the Fourth Class. On the arrival of my Imperial Emblem be it known to you that the British Embassy has reported and requested as follows:
>
> The Prince of Wales, son of the Queen of England, manifested the wish that my imperial government should be pleases to concede as a gift, a piece of ground of ten thousand square 'zirae' approximately for the establishment by the English members of the Society of St. John at Jerusalem of a Hospice and a place for tending gratuitously poor invalids.
>
> Such an establishment being one of public utility, it was decided in my council of ministers that a piece of ground of the extent required should be granted in the same manner and under the same condition [as] the one which was previously granted there to the Prince of Prussia for the foundation of a similar establishment by the German branch of the said society, and at a place free of all local objections; upon this, my Imperial sanction having been besought, I was pleased to grant it and to convey it through this my noble Firman emanating from my Imperial Divan, and delivered to whom it may concern.
>
> You, therefore, who are the above-mentioned Governor, have to provide for the required piece of ground of ten thousands 'zirae' approximately, and one which may not give rise to local objections, and to show and offer the said ground

> to the aforesaid English Society, while taking care that it should be employed in the manner and under conditions identical to those under which the grant of such piece of ground to the German branch of the Society was previously made. 299 Djeazil Lakhir (24th April 1882).[44]

Dr Thomas Chaplin took part in the initiative to ease eye diseases in Jerusalem, by serving as an Honorary Associate of the Council of the Order of St. John of Jerusalem. He participated in a meeting on July 7, 1882 in the Jerusalem Chamber of Westminster Abbey, held by the Order of St. John in London, in the presence of Edmund Lechmere. At this meeting speeches were delivered concerning the importance of constructing a hospital and clinic for eye diseases in Jerusalem. It was resolved to dispatch Dr G. S. Waddell, then assistant surgeon at the Eye and Ear Hospital in Shrewsbury, to be the doctor of the hospital that would be opened in Jerusalem.[45] Waddell arrived in the city on December 1882 and immediately set to treating scores of patients daily in his temporary clinic in Jerusalem. According to his reports, within six months, he treated 1,952 patients, and another 3,200 received some advice and medicine. On average, 80 patients daily received treatment, and on some days the physician was seeing 140 patients. Waddell returned to England in 1884 because of illness and was succeeded by Dr John Hovell Ogilvie.[46]

The firman that was given to the Order in April 1882 was useful, especially when Dr Chaplin found a suitable plot of land for the Ophthalmic Hospital. The chosen site, on which a large house was obtained by purchase, was situated east of the Bethlehem Road, bounded from the east by the Valley of Hinnom, not far from the Jaffa gate. The building stood on the west end of the plot, had a good water supply, was 'extremely well built of the best materials' and contained eighteen chambers (today it houses the Har-Zion Hotel on 17 Hebron Road).[47]

The hospital began operation in early 1883.[48] However, the official inauguration was in November 1886. Sir Edmund Lechmere, General Secretary of the Order, and Lady Lechmere visited Jerusalem and the hospital, and were the honorary guests at the ceremony, along with other distinguished visitors such as the

Governor of Jerusalem, the Greek Orthodox Patriarch, the Armenian Patriarch and the Jewish Chief Rabbi. The latter presented a memorial in Hebrew, recording the gratitude of the members of the Jewish community and their 'confidence in the absence of any proselytising'.[49]

Since a Turkish regulation required hospitals in Jerusalem to be attached to a specific church, to enable them to receive drugs and other medical supplies free of import taxes, the British Ambassador in Constantinople made a successful effort to get this privilege directly to the Order. The patients arrived from all over the Middle East, and belonged to all ethnic groups and religious faiths; all patients were treated free of charge by the physicians and the resident surgeon, John Ogilvie.[50]

Ogilvie's successor was Dr Cant who arrived in Jerusalem in April 1889, after obtaining a permit in Constantinople to work as a physician all over the Ottoman Empire. He acted as medical superintendent, and served in the hospital for 23 years. Cant reported on thousands of patients and hundreds of operations. The number of beds increased to sixteen, which were always full. In 1890 the institution treated 9,468 patients out of which 3,757 were new cases. In 1894 a house for the physician and a new outpatient block was built in memory of General Gordon. In 1897 the workload increased so much that the hospital was unable to cope with the needs of the city population.[51]

George Francis Popham Blyth, bishop of Jerusalem, wrote to the Prince of Wales in September 28, 1901, attesting to the hospital's activity:

> I am glad that the Order of St. John has been able to give great prominence to the Ophthalmic Hospital, of which of which you are Chairman. It is doing excellent work, and it is known and trusted throughout the country, and even to Moab and the Trans-Jordan country.
>
> Dr. Cant's name is one of the note here. He performed an operation for cataract on me last year, quite painlessly and quite successfully. I must have resigned otherwise, but I can now see forty miles of distance and read 'diamond type'. I heard of him in England as one of the first men of the day, to

whom anything might be opened at home. I only got the same attention that he gave to an old bedridden woman who was his patient before me. He is in every way a good man, but very retiring.

The work of the hospital is sometimes spoken against because it is not directly missionary. But, it is known far and wide as the work of charity and philanthropy by men who do the work for the sake of Christ. It is neither mixed up with proselytism (as our missions have been much) nor with politics (as foreign institutions are), but it has done a fine work in breaking down prejudice, and it is real and thorough. The new building will be a great advantage. It is well that the ancient Order should have its hospital here, accessible to all, and free. It has greatly subdued the worst forms of eye diseases, as people now understand that their sight can be saved if they go in time.[52]

In April 1911, Dr Cant was replaced by Dr Edwin Ward who died a short time afterward. Cant returned to Palestine and his former position, to replace Dr Ward until Dr D. Heron arrived. Heron stayed in the job until December 25, 1914, when the hospital was closed due to the First World War. During the War, the St. John's Hospital was commandeered by Turkish soldiers who turned the building into a barracks.[53] When the British army entered Jerusalem in 1917, the structure became the headquarters of the British officer Major General Shea. On February 26, 1919, the hospital was renovated, and reopened in a rededication ceremony in the presence of General Edmund Allenby (1861-1936) himself. Colonel Dr John Strathearn was appointed to run the hospital, serving in this capacity until 1941.[54]

German Templars' Hospital in Jaffa

In the mid-nineteenth century, in the Kingdom of Württemberg in southwestern Germany, a religious movement arose and tried to introduce reforms in the Protestant Church. Out of this 'Pietistic' movement, emerged the 'Templar Society'. The members of this association were extreme in their criticism of the church establishment, and were finally expelled from its ecclesiastical ranks.

In 1868 the society decided to realize the 'Gathering of the People of God' in Jerusalem and sent its two founders to the Holy Land. During the fifty years of German settlement in Palestine under Turkish rule, seven German colonies were established: in Haifa and Jaffa (both in 1869): Sarona (today the heart of Tel Aviv, in 1871), and the 'Refaim' colony outside the walls of Jerusalem (in 1873). At the beginning of the twentieth century, the second generation of settlers established three more colonies: Wilhelma near Ben-Gurion airport (today Bnei-Atarot, in 1902), Bethlehem Galilee in the north of the country (in 1906), and the next-door German colony of Waldheim (today Alonei Abba, in 1907).[55]

As noted above, in 1869 the Templers established their second colony north of the city of Jaffa (today at the corner of Eilat and Auerbach Streets in Tel Aviv). The settlers bought a number of prefabricated wooden houses, remains of the colony that had been established by American settlers from Maine, United States, that was abandoned in 1867.[56] When the German settlers arrived in Jaffa, there were no doctors at the level of European standards in the city. Since it was a port city and the main gateway for those coming to the Land of Israel, the only medical services provided by the authorities was limited to a quarantine station to check the health of those arriving from abroad. The only doctors, until the arrival of the Templars, were those of the quarantine station whose medical knowledge, acquired locally, was of a far lower level than the knowledge acquired in European universities. Their medical activities were limited to bloodletting, suction cups and leeches.[57]

The modest medical enterprise in the city of Jaffa, which eventually developed into a modern hospital belonging to the Templar Society, was initiated by two men. The first was Peter Martin Metzler (1824-1907), a German missionary who had been sent in 1853 to Palestine by a Mission Society in Basle, in order to promote business initiatives that would support the physical presence and activities of the missionaries.[58] Five years after his arrival in Jerusalem, Metzler came to Jaffa, and by order of the head of his Mission, engaged in trade and even set up a small hostel in his house. At the beginning of the 1860s he made the acquaintance of one of his visitors, the Russian baron, Plato von Ustinov (1840-1918), the grandfather of the late Sir Peter Ustinov (1921-2004), who financed the establishment of a pharmacy within the city of Jaffa in 1863.[59]

After their arrival, the Templars rented two rooms near Metzler's pharmacy and treated their own patients as well as a few non-Templar patients. The modest clinic, which in those days contained six beds, was managed by the Templar physician, Dr Gottlob David Sandel (1817-1879), who had arrived from Germany in 1870. A year later the Templars established their third colony of Sarona, near Jaffa on the banks of Wadi Musrara (today the Ayalon River in the heart of Tel Aviv). The wadi, which contained stagnant water, was a source of infection and caused an increase in the number of sick people among the Templars. Their health declined to such an extent that many of them died of malaria and typhus.[60] Sandel therefore decided in 1874 to expand the clinic in Jaffa into a small hospital and to establish it in the heart of the German colony in Jaffa. Thus, in that year, the new medical institution was set up in a private home in the colony donated by one of the settlers, and already had ten hospital beds. A few doctors worked at this hospital until the end of the decade. Samuel Hoffmann, a medical student and the son of the founder of the Templar Society, arrived in 1874 from Germany, and began to serve under Sandel. When Hoffmann completed his training in Jaffa, he was appointed as medical director of the German Deaconesses of Kaiserwerth Hospital in Jerusalem. Carl Lorch (1851-1928) assisted in the hospital and served as a male nurse. Lorch was even sent, at the recommendation of Sandel, to study medicine in Erlangen in Germany, and later he returned to Palestine. In 1878 Dr Franz Gottlieb Paulus (1849-1919) was appointed as director of the hospital instead of Sandel, who died a year later.

In 1878 the Templars transferred their management centre from Jaffa to the new colony that had been established in Emek Refaim in Jerusalem. Their school was also transferred, and Paulus then transferred his hospital to the vacated wooden structure. Although this structure had a few deficiencies, it allowed for the expansion and development of the medical institution and it served the Templars and the settlers in the surrounding area until the Second World War.[61]

The hospital suffered from financial difficulties in most of the years it functioned, and the Templars tried to overcome this difficulty by instituting a system of medical insurance. Every German settler set aside a certain annual sum for the hospital, according to the amount set by the heads of the Templar Society, and in exchange they received free medical treatment whenever necessary. In 1902, for example, the insurance rates were as follows: A family of up to five members – 24 francs per year; for every additional member of the family – another 4 francs; after 50 days of hospitalization – 2.5 francs per extra day; for a non-insured patient – 4 francs per day.[62] In 1878, the Russian baron, von Ustinov who had in the meantime immigrated to the Land of Israel and taken up residence in a building that he had bought in the German colony in Jaffa, provided assistance to the medical institution. He established a Rehabilitation centre at his home near the hospital, in which 22 patients from the German colonies and other patients from around the country were rehabilitated. At the same time he financed the full cost of three hospital beds at his home.[63]

In 1880 Paulus left the hospital in Jaffa, worked for a time in Jerusalem, and then returned to Germany. Carl Lorch, who had in the meantime completed his training abroad, returned to Palestine and directed the hospital in Jaffa for 47 years (1880-1927). In 1886 the Templars constructed a new wing of the hospital financed by von Ustinov and a number of other German institutions. The hospital now contained four additional spacious wards. Another initiative of von Ustinov was to buy land to build a new modern hospital that was to have been erected between the German colony in Jaffa and the sister colony of Sarona. The ceremonial laying of the cornerstone was held in April 1913. But the First World War, which broke out a year later, changed the entire situation and the institution was never built. A short while later von Ustinov left Palestine and died in 1918.[64]

The German hospital also provided services to the Arab residents of Jaffa and the surrounding areas. Sometimes, especially after the wave of immigration of the early 1880s, even the Jews of Jaffa and the Jewish colonies benefited from its services. From the data amassed over 42 years (1885-1927) it seems that 26% of the patients were not Templars. Between 1885 and 1927, 2305 patients were hospitalized for 35,869 days, and 129 died in the hospital.[65]

Scottish Hospital (EMMS) in Nazareth

Dr Kaloost P. Vartan (1835-1908), a physician of Turkish Armenian origin, was the initiator of the Scottish medical mission in Nazareth. In 1861 he was appointed by the 'London Jews Society for Sending Aid to the Protestants of Syria' as its medical emissary to the Middle East. That society was established after the massacre of Arab Christians in Syria and Lebanon during the civil war of 1860. Prior to his position in Nazareth, Vartan had served as an interpreter for the British army during the Crimean war, studied medicine in England and Scotland (Edinburgh) on a scholarship of the Edinburgh Medical Missionary Society (EMMS) and became a member of the Church of England. He was given £100 and an outfit allowance and was sent to Beirut.[66] Soon after arriving, Vartan decided not to get involved in a dispute in Beirut, between Catholics and Protestants concerning the civil war. Subsequently he was asked to open a dispensary in Nazareth, and in 1861 he joined Johannes Zeller, a missionary of the CMS in Nazareth, and began practicing medicine.[67]

The local healers in Nazareth objected to the modern physician, and were afraid that their customers would prefer his services. These healers conducted a campaign of slanders against Vartan. However, he continued to practice in his clinic in town, fortified his professional status and gained the trust of the local inhabitants. In 1865 he treated the son of the mayor of Nazareth, and won the title 'The Great Doctor'.[68]

The Committee that sent Vartan to Nazareth was dissolved in 1864, which left him without a source of funds. For two years he was supported privately by Dr Burns Thomson, the superintendent of the Coogate dispensary. Vartan was later nominated by the EMMS directors as their agent in Nazareth and secured his annual salary (£100) for two years commencing January 1866. The same year he was invited to Edinburgh for discussions with the heads of the mission and for the purpose of his post-graduate studies. During that visit he tried to raise funds for building a hospital in Nazareth, but was not successful. He returned to the Holy Land with Miss Mary Anna Stewart, a Scottish nurse he married in June 1867.[69]

At first Dr Vartan received patients in an improvised dispensary in the house in which he lived. In 1867, he installed eight beds for surgical cases in a large room he rented near the Maronite Church in town. In three years he treated 36 inpatients per day, as well as an average of 85 outpatients.[70] At the same time he operated a Sunday school and a medical school in Nazareth following the programme of Edinburgh Medical School and the American University in Beirut. He chose seven students and taught them for two years. Eventually, the programme was terminated due to lack of funds.[71]

Vartan received permission from the EMMS to acquire a piece of land for the hospital. However, eventually he managed only to rent such plots and intended to build a hospital and residence for himself there.[72] After some years the rented site was too small and inadequate to serve as a hospital and accordingly in 1879 he bought a plot of 35 acres overlooking Nazareth.[73] In 1880, Vartan visited England and raised £3,000 for building the hospital. Two years later, after a long period of providing medical treatment in an unsuitable environment, he decided to build the new hospital. He laid the foundation stone in April 4, 1882.[74] Vartan was convinced that he would get a firman from the Turkish authorities, but he had been misled. The land and the modern unfinished building were taken by the authorities, paying a mere £1,000 as compensation. This building was completed after Vartan's death, and was never used as a hospital. It was used by the Turks during the First World War as a police headquarter and is known today in Nazareth as *Kishle* (Prison).[75]

In 1895 the directors of the EMMS directed Dr Vartan to buy other premises. However this was delayed due to his illness and his leave in Scotland. After his return, in 1903 he started to search for a new site, with the help of Dr Frederick John Scrimgeour who was sent for his assistance from Damascus. In 1905, they rented a house in the centre of town and operated it as a temporary hospital. In 1906, a suitable site on a hillside west of the town was found and purchased. The firman was easily obtained this time. However, Vartan died on December 3, 1908 and never saw the completion of his new building.[76] Dr Vartan practiced as a physician in Nazareth and its vicinity for 47 years as a missionary among the Arabs. He was the first modern physician, and for ten years the only one between Jerusalem and Beirut.[77] He was succeeded by Dr Scrimgeour who continued operating the rented premises in town.

A review of this modest institution was given by the Scottish Reverend W. Ewing during his second visit to the Holy Land in 1912. He described Scrimgeour, the emissary of the EMMS, and his wish to practice in a modern hospital that he hoped would be built on a commanding position in the city. However, when Ewing visited the mission, Scrimgeour worked 'amid many hampering conditions', in a hired native house that was 'crumbling to ruin'.[78] But even in that facility, the medical work was carried out properly. According to Dr Vartan's yearly report of 1898, the medical mission supplied 8427 consultations with prescriptions (7702 in 1897); of these 5743 were treated in the dispensary, 2684 were treated in their homes. 5747 were Christians and 2680 were Muslims.[79] A variety of treatments were performed in the hospital. For example, in the report of 1906 one can learn that the following operations took place: abscesses – 250; amputations – 6; calculus of bladder – 5; cysts – 5; curettings – 4; diseases of bone – 40; circumcision – 8; glands – 18; sinuses and fistulae – 42; gunshots 7; tonsils and adenoids – 8; removal of foreign bodies – 11; hernia – 1; gynaecological operations – 4; tumours – 17; Lister's excision of wrist – 1; Thiersch skin-grafting – 2; various – 78; laparotomies – 2; radical cure of hydrocele – 3; eye operations – 29; iridectomy – 4; cataract – 4; ectropion – 4; evisceration – 1; various (eye diseases) 32. Total – 586.[80]

Scrimgeour only managed to inaugurate the doctor's house in 1912. The building of the hospital was almost complete but due to the outbreak of the First World War, the British physicians had to leave Palestine and the medical institution was closed.[81] It was only in April 25, 1924 that EMMS inaugurated a modern hospital in Nazareth (in Diana St. 11/13 of today).[82]

Scottish Hospital in Tiberias

The sanitary conditions in the city of Tiberias were very poor and the inhabitants suffered from various diseases and epidemics every few years. There was no system of sewage and the cesspools that were attached to the houses were seldom cleaned. No wells or water cisterns existed and the water was drawn straight from the lake. The shores of the lake were full of 'ash heaps and dunghills', the water was impure and unfit for drinking. Malaria and dysentery were very common and the mortality among children was very high.[83] After the cholera epidemic hit the city in 1865, the Jewish community established a society that started to raise funds to build a hospital. The building was constructed, but since the society could not find a physician, the building was used as a shelter for elderly people. From time to time, visiting physicians supplied services to the inhabitants of Tiberias.[84]

In 1883, James H. Wilson (1837-1925) of the 'Sea of Galilee Mission' of the Free Church of Scotland visited the Holy Land for six weeks.[85] He was asked by the Jewish Mission Committee of his Church to look for any opening for carrying 'something for Israel in their own land' into effect. His inquiries in Jerusalem convinced him that the field of mission in Palestine was fully occupied. 'It almost seemed as if Christian agencies of many kinds were standing in each other's way' wrote Wilson. After inspecting the Christian, mainly Protestant activity in other cities in the Holy Land, the Jewish Mission Committee chose to operate either in Safed or in Tiberias.[86]

In February 1884 Dr David Watt Torrance (1862-1923) left Scotland for the Holy Land. Torrance, a Scot, had completed his medical studies in Glasgow in 1883, and a year later joined the medical missionary team of the Free Church of Scotland.[87] As the missionary elected physician, he had to find out the best area, between the Northern towns of Safed and Tiberias, for a new Medical Mission to the Jews. His companions were James Wells (1838-1909) of Glasgow, Convener of the Jewish Mission Committee, Dr R. Laidlaw, superintendent of Glasgow Medical Mission and Dr Vartan of Nazareth. The delegation visited both cities, and since the London Jews Society already had a mission station in Safed, their recommendation was Tiberias. In their report to the Jewish Mission Committee in Scotland they listed the reasons for establishing a medical mission in the town. They wrote that there was a great need for a doctor in Tiberias and that no qualified physician resided there. Several of the Jews they met assured them that 'a European doctor would be greatly prized among them, as they all felt that he was very much needed, both for the inhabitants and the bathers [pilgrims in the lake]'.[88] It was the same recommendation that had been made by Robert Murray M'Cheyne (1813-1843) and Andrew Alexander Bonar (1810-1892), the emissaries of the Church of Scotland on their visit to the Holy Land forty-five years earlier.[89] The first month after Torrance's arrival spent with Dr Kaloost Vartan of Nazareth taught him much, including 'the unhealthiness of the place, the fanatical nature of the inhabitants, Jewish and Muslims'.[90] Torrance started to practice medicine before a stock of medications could arrive from Scotland. Since it was further detained in Trieste, he managed to find some old drugs in the town, such as Epsom salts and castor oil. During those early days Torrance bought a piece of land in the Northern part of town near the ruins of the Crusader wall, for his planned hospital. Until approval of a firman by the Turkish Authorities, he rented a building in town with the help of a donation from Scotland. He renovated the building as a hospital, with wards for men and women and an operating room.[91]

The arrival of Torrance, the Scottish physician and missionary, in Tiberias, encouraged the Jewish community to try to establish its own medical services. Among the Jewish physicians who practiced in the city was the well known Dr Hillel Yaffe (1864-1936). Arriving in Palestine in 1890, he accepted the offer from the *Ashkenazi* Jewish community in Tiberias and came to town in 1891 accompanied by a pharmacist. Yaffe renovated a house near the city wall and started to practice free of charge. His stay was successful and he was even appointed as a municipal physician, but, in 1893 he left to establish a hospital in the young Jewish settlement of Zichron Yaakov.[92] The various Jewish physicians who kept practicing in Tiberias during the years, usually sent their severe cases to the Scottish hospital to be treated, advised or operated on by Dr Torrance. He became the highest medical authority in the Northern part of the Holy Land at that time.

In the spring of 1893 a ceremony for digging the first sod to prepare the ground for building the upcoming hospital was performed, and the Turkish governor publicly read the firman. The inauguration itself took place on January 1, 1894. The new hospital contained 24 beds and six cots, instead of the desired 60 beds. There was a dispensary department attached to it, in which 40-50 patients were treated daily. The hospital was closed in the hottest summer months, but the dispensary remained open.[93] The main entrance to the hospital grounds was on the south side facing town and the hospital itself, an oblong grey-stone building, faced the lake. The dispensary and its waiting-room were at the southern end. On the second floor was the male ward, containing eight beds, two cots, a male attendant's room and private room with two beds. The southern part of the grounds was occupied by the female ward, containing eight beds and two cots.[94] The hospital provided medical services for the large population of the Jordan Valley and the Galilee. Figures concerning number of patients were given frequently by Torrance. For example, in 9 months between October 1907 and June 1908, 366 patients were in-patients. Of the out-patients, 7,284 were seen in the Consulting Room, and 13,915 were seen in the Surgical Dressing-Room. During that period 625 operations were carried out.[95]

Dr Torrance died in August 1923 and was buried in the hospital grounds on the shore of the Sea of Galillee. His son, Dr Herbert Torrance (1892-1977) who joined his father in 1921, continued to work in Tiberias until his retirement in 1953. Altogether father and son served the people of the Galilee for 70 years.

The hospital in Tiberias, as did other mission hospitals, had a missionary aspect as well. From one of the descriptions of its medical staff and achievements, in the Free Church of Scotland's journal, one can learn about the difficulties of medical mission work in the Tiberias Hospital. Dr Ernest Muir, a Scottish medical missionary, reported the scepticism among many patients during their stay in the hospital:

> 'As one of them enters the dispensary for the first time, you can see on his face that he distrusts you. He thinks that you

wish to take advantage of him, and he watches every movement you make with suspicion. When he leaves the hospital one or two weeks later, the change is wonderful. He suspects you no more and his distrust has given place to gratitude'. Regarding the slow process Muir added: 'This slow, leavening process, which has been going on for many years, is telling for good on the people, and, though it be but slowly, yet advance is being made'.[96]

Dismantling of the Anglo-Prussian Bishopric

Samuel Gobat, the second Protestant Bishop in Jerusalem, died on May 11, 1879. A month later, Benjamin Disraeli (1804-1881) proposed the appointment of Joseph Barclay (1831-1881) as the next Bishop in Jerusalem. Barclay had served in the 1860s as Head of the London Jews Society in Palestine. After some hesitations, Barclay agreed to accept the position, and on February 3, 1880, he entered the gates of the Holy City. But he never had the chance of leaving his imprint on the missionary work in the country. On October 22, 1881, Barclay died in Jerusalem following a brief illness and was buried, like his predecessors, in the Protestant cemetery on Mount Zion.

Immediately after Barclay's demise, rumors began to spread that Germany had no intention of appointing a successor to the late Bishop. The focus of German dissatisfaction was their sense that within the framework of the Bishopric, the German Protestant community in the Holy Land was disadvantaged in comparison to its British counterpart.[97] The German community was not felt to be a full partner in shaping the lifestyle of the Protestants in Jerusalem and was particularly disadvantaged in the prayer schedules at 'Christ Church', which belonged to the London Jews Society. This inequality was especially noticeable in a period when Bishop Gobat, who had been chosen by the Prussians, was obviously expected to look after the community who had sent him. During these years the feeling of being excluded festered in the hearts of members of the Evangelical Church in Palestine, and later, after German prestige grew in Europe and the status of the Germans in the Holy Land was flourishing, these sentiments were exacerbated. The negotiations between Britain and Germany, which began in July 1882 in order to settle the delicate balance of power within the joint organization of the Jerusalem Bishopric, lasted a number of years. The breakup of the Anglo-Prussian Bishopric in 1887 led to the establishment of two separate institutions. Germany founded the Evangelical Bishopric, with its centre in the compound of the 'Church of the Redeemer' near the 'Holy Sepulchre' in Jerusalem, whereas the British set up a similar institution in the Anglican 'St. George College' in Jerusalem.

Among the historians analyzing the nineteenth century there is a widespread belief that competition between the European Powers promoted the modernization process in the Land of Israel. Emphasis was placed on the struggle between the Protestant Church to which England and Germany were affiliated, the Catholics who were identified with France and Austria, and the Orthodox Church identified with Russia. Less attention was given to the competition between Protestant England and Germany. In the beginning of their settlement attempts in the Land of Israel these two nations cooperated in establishing a joint bishopric, while in the medical sphere the German institutions received the assistance of British physicians in Palestine. Yet over the course of time, mainly after Germany became united in the framework of the Second Reich, this cooperation acquired a competitive aspect and each acted within the narrow framework of its own hospitals.

Catholic Medical Activity, Institutions and Politics

Unlike its sister powers, France had maintained a continuous presence in the Land of Israel ever since the first trade agreement (capitulation) signed between the King of France and the Turkish Sultan in 1535. This agreement enabled France to ensure its position as a defender of Christianity, granting protection to all Christians in the Ottoman Empire and in Palestine in particular, without distinction of nationality. In this way it gained preferred status over other European states. After the establishment of the Anglo-Prussian bishopric, and the increase of interest in the Holy Land, France made energetic attempts to fortify its standing as the foremost European power in the Land of Israel. To its chagrin, the other powers also increased their activities in the country and tried to rid themselves of patronage by French nationals and institutions.

The establishment of the Anglo-Prussian bishopric at the beginning of the 1840s prompted the French to take action. The establishment of this influential Christian institution, which was given the support and blessing of prominent personalities in Europe at that time, induced influential circles in the Catholic world to demand that the Pope appoint a Vatican Representative as a counterweight to the Protestant Bishop. When Samuel Gobat was elected as the Second Protestant Bishop in Jerusalem in 1846, and began to work among the Christian Arabs in the country, the Pope hurriedly revived the Catholic Patriarchate, the first since Crusader times. From the time that the Latin Patriarch was appointed, the number of French institutions increased in the country. It is worth mentioning mainly the hostel of Notre-Dame de France and the adjoining hospital of Saint Louis. These two buildings were erected in the vicinity of the impressive Russian building complex in the 'Russian Compound' which had most probably prompted the French to make their own display of wealth and distinction.

Nevertheless, once the powers had established their own Consulates, they no longer needed the services of France. In this way a bitter struggle began that lasted throughout the century over the validity of the French 'protectorate'. After France lost its status as the defender of Orthodox and Protestant foreign nationals, it asserted its right to grant protection to all the Catholic institutions even if their members were the subjects of other states. By the end of the nineteenth century no one could recall the real meaning of the French protectorate.

French Hospital of Saint Louis

Dr Arnold Mendelssohn (d. 1864), a Prussian Protestant and the grandson of the Jewish philosopher Moses Mendelssohn (1729-1786), established the French Catholic hospital in Jerusalem. Mendelssohn arrived in the Holy City as a British subject in June 1851 and tried to practice medicine in the English mission hospital directed by Dr Edward Macgowan. Disappointed by the fact that he did not succeed in private practice as well, he acquired a French citizenship in order to join a French-protected medical institution in town. Mendelssohn, together with the French Consul in Palestine and an Italian priest, managed to obtain the financials means to procure a private house, near the Khan of the Copts in Jerusalem.[98]

On November 1, 1851 the new Catholic hospital was inaugurated, named after Louis IX (1215-1270) the leader of the fifth crusade, and having 22 beds and a dispensary.[99] The new medical institution was operated by the Sisters of St. Joseph de l'Apparition. Several months after the opening, Mendelssohn and the French Consul in Jerusalem, Paul Emile Botta (1802-1870), managed to claim Giuseppe Valerga (1813-1827), the Latin Patriarch in the town, as the hospital's patron.[100]

The Patriarch and the French Consul tried to find a location for a new and improved hospital and in 1868 moved into the former complex of the French Consulate.[101] The hospital continued to serve both the interests of the French government and the Latin Patriarch, and the French Consul Botta continued to supply a yearly sum of 12,000 francs for the hospital. The name of the hospital was changed several times and finally in 1871 it became Hôpital Saint Louis.

The French Baron Marie Paul Ame'de'e de Piellat (1852-1925) was one of the most important figures behind the establishment of French Catholic medical institution in Jerusalem. On his first visit to the Holy Land in 1874, as a devout Catholic he felt both impressed and threatened by the institutions that were built and operated by the Protestants under the German and English protection, and the Orthodox institution under Russian protection. A few years later, in 1876, de Piellat made his second visit to Palestine, accompanied by his mother. Both acted efficiently for the benefit of the small hospital of Saint Louis, which was situated in the internal plaza of Jaffa Gate and operated in a high density population and with inadequate medical instruments.[102]

In 1878 the Baron and his mother acquired a large piece of land outside the city walls, across the north-west corner of the city, opposite the New Gate. The cornerstone was laid on May 4, 1879 by the Latin Patriarch. On January 1, 1882, the hospital was opened and was operated by the nuns of Soeurs de Saint Joseph de l'Apparition, who also ran the old Catholic hospital. The Baron financed the lower level of the hospital, including a chapel for the nuns and another larger chapel for the patients and the general public. He himself decorated and painted this floor mainly with crusaders' symbols and scenes. The hospital was meant to treat the Catholic French pilgrims who de Piellat intended to bring to the Holy Land, and to serve the general public at other times. Indeed the hospital did help the Arab population in Jerusalem, Muslims as well as Christian. De Piellat continued to support the hospital and to keep it modern and updated.[103]

Order of St. John of God's Hospital (Tantur)

The Catholic order of St. John of God started to operate in the Holy Land as early as 1857 with a mobile hospital that traveled among the Bedouins.[104]

The Austrian Consul in Jerusalem, Bernard Graf Caboga-Cerva (1823-1882) who was a member of the Order of the Knights of Malta, arrived in the city in 1867. One of his first actions was to raise funds from friends all over the world, and to purchase, on June 4, 1869, the hilltop of Tantur. The plot of land, formerly donated in 1110 by crusading King Baldwin to the order of St. John, was located south of Jerusalem on the road to Bethlehem.[105] Caboga registered the place under his name, paying 32, 206 piaster, and built a small tower for his frequent use.[106]

The Austrian Kaiser Franz Josef (1830-1916) visited Palestine in November 1869, during his voyage for the opening ceremony of the Suez Canal. He paid a visit to the site of Tantur and heard from Caboga his plans for a hospital. Upon his return to Vienna, the Kaiser sent a donation of 50,000 franks and ordered his chancellor to promote the Jerusalem project. Accordingly Caboga began to build a number of rooms near the tower and in 1874 he already had a clinic with 7 beds.[107]

A firman for erecting a permanent hospital was issued by the Sultan on March 4, 1876 in a ceremony conducted on the hill. On that occasion the premises were transferred to the Bohemian Priorate of Malta which had built the hospital of the Sovereign Military Order of Malta, inaugurated on June 11, 1876.[108] The hospital was two stories high; each floor had long promenading porticos arched open to the fresh air. It faced east to receive the morning light and to keep the afternoon sun at its back. The large towers of three floors were situated on both sides of the building (north and south), and a chapel was built on the north side as well. In the front of the hospital, around the old tower, there were gardens of fruit trees and Jerusalem pines.[109]

Caboga had to assemble the medical staff himself and he handed over the management of the institution to the Brothers of the Bavarian Province of the Hospitaller Order of St. John of God. Their German leader, Dr Othmar Mayer, soon had arguments with Caboga, who served as an administrator of the Hospice. Due to international political issues and events between Austria and Germany the period of cooperation in Tantur was brief. In 1880, Othmar Mayer left the institution and two years later Caboga died.

In 1890 the medical institution of Tantur was again under Austrian authority, with the management of the Austrian Province of Graz, and in two years six beds were added to the hospital.[110] In 1894 the Brothers of the Hospitaller Order returned to practice in the hospital. They enlarged the facilities in 1902-3, and constructed a new wing in 1909. In a confidential economic report written by Heinrich Jehlitschka (b.1861), the Austrian Consul in Jerusalem in April 20, 1899, he mentioned that the hospital at Tantur treated 14,000 patients each year.[111] During the First World War the hospital served sick and injured German and Austrian soldiers. After the war the hospital underwent a slow demise until the Second World War, when the British requisitioned Tantur and used it as an internment camp for Italian missionaries in Palestine.[112]

Austrian Hospital in Nazareth

Dr Othmar Mayer, the German physician, and pharmacists left Tantur in December 1880 and tried to open a hospital in Bethlehem. In 1881 he settled in Nazareth, rented a house and started to operate a small hospital and a dispensary. He received a donation of 800 florins from the Austrian Crown Prince, Rudolph von Habsburg (1858-1889) to build a permanent hospital in Nazareth. (It is possible that the Crown Prince gave that donation due to a severe attack of malaria he experienced after visiting the Holy Land and Nazareth in 1881). Mayer himself made a fundraising tour in Europe and returned in March 1882 with almost 9000 Lire. The inauguration of the hospital in the rented house took place on March 16, 1882. Although it was a small institution with six beds, more than 3434 patients were treated there before the end of the year, about half Catholics and the rest Muslims.[113]

Dr Philip Benito Wagner (d. 1882), a German physician and a surgeon, joined the newly established Nazareth hospital in July 1882. Just before he died, Wagner purchased out of his private resources, a large plot of land on a hill outside the city (on Namsawi St. of today). On November 1882 Mayar began to build a modest hospital with four beds on the hill and inaugurated it in November 1884. The hospital's name was 'Krankenhaus zur Heiligen Familie' (The Hospital of the Holy Family) containing at that time 10 beds. Disputes between the German physicians of the hospital and the Franciscans, who felt their hold in Nazareth was threatened by German nationals, led to violent actions against Mayer on February 21, 1889. Soon after, the hospital was closed, the Germans were expelled and the French mercenaries occupied the hospital.[114]

Several attempts to re-open the hospital failed until June 1893, when the Austrians, Dr Petrus Damian Amschel and Dr Johannes Berchmans, were again sent to renovate and open the hospital. The medical institution suffered from financial difficulties and only one of the planned buildings was partly built, on the road from Nazareth to Tiberias, containing 30 beds. The other part of the plot was sold to relieve the financial problems.

During the First World War the hospital was confiscated by the Turks and served as a military hospital. As late as 1959 a small modern hospital was built on the same site, operated by the Italian Lombard-Venetian province and having the same name - Ospedale Sacra Famiglia.[115]

Orthodox Medical Activity, Institutions and Politics

During the first half of the nineteenth century, Czarist Russia enjoyed a special status in the Holy Land. Although Catholic France was considered the protector of Christianity in the Land of Israel, Russia had two outstanding advantages that ensured her standing. The first one that characterized her activities and gave her an advantage over the other European powers was the size of the Orthodox community under her protection, most of whom were Arab Christians. At the beginning of the nineteenth century, when the European powers began searching for wards to be taken under their protection so that their standing would be enhanced, the Orthodox community already numbered 20,000, constituting 90 per cent of all the Arab Christians in the country. The second advantage came from the mass Russian pilgrimages that annually visited the holy places in the Land of Israel. Thousands of pilgrims, zealous and enthusiastic, who arrived at the Holy Sepulchre at Easter to take part in the ceremony of the 'Holy Fire', crammed the streets of Jerusalem. In their long journey, the pilgrims were accommodated in poor Greek Orthodox Monasteries, and suffered from the effects of malnutrition, bad sanitation and the physical demands of an unfamiliar climate. With no medical aid, many died on the way, and those that reached the Holy Land were mostly exhausted and sick.[116]

The hegemony at the beginning of the nineteenth century made Russia so complacent that it did nothing to fortify its already strong standing. Russia therefore found herself, by the middle of the century, lagging behind in the race for European prestige in the Holy Land. At the end of the Crimean War (1853-1856), which had broken out over disputes regarding the holy places between Orthodox priests under Russian protection and Catholic priests under French protection, Russia found herself defeated on the battlefield, which also injured her standing in the Land of Israel. Russia therefore began to adopt a more aggressive policy in order to strengthen its weakened position. A religious commission that arrived in Jerusalem to represent Russian interests in general, purchased in 1859 the *Maidan* compound, the Turkish parade grounds north of the Old City, and began to erect upon it the 'New Jerusalem'. Within this compound, which was surrounded by a wall, monumental buildings were constructed at the beginning of the 1860s to include hostels for men and women, a Consulate and a church. In order to serve the thousands of pilgrims (over 10,000 at the end of the nineteenth century) who came to the Land of Israel during each year, and to serve the needs of the Orthodox community in Jerusalem, a hospital was also built within the Russian compound.

Russian Pilgrims' Hospital

The hospital was planned according to the model of the Dutch hospital in Ismir and was approved by the Russian Ministry of Health in 1860.[117] The hospital was inaugurated in 1862 (in the 'Russian compound' of today) and contained an operating theatre and 30 beds in 2 large rooms for the patients, premises for the physician and pharmacist, a room for the nurses, a laboratory, a storage room and a workshop.[118] In 1872, the hospital contained 60 beds, and by 1887 it contained 75 beds. In 1887, the Hospital of the German Deaconesses of Kaiserswerth had 40 beds; the France Hôpital Saint Louis had 32 beds; the English Mission Hospital had 27 beds; the Greek Hospital had 24 beds; the Bikkur Holim hospital had 25 beds; the Hôpital Israelite Mayer Rothschild had 18 beds. According to these figures the Russian hospital was the largest in Jerusalem at the time.[119]

The number of patients who were hospitalized was dependant on the varying numbers of pilgrims, and increased every year between December and May. The hospital also accepted non-Russians in small numbers, primarily Christian-Arabs; however, very few Jews were recorded.[120] The medical supplies and medicines were shipped from France and were of the best quality. The hospital possessed modern surgical equipment and apparatus for blood transfusion and stomach lavage. The medical staff included about 14 professionals, a physician (who acted a director as well), surgeon, pharmacists and a few practical 'nurses' and helpers. The nursing staff were not qualified or well trained, although they worked very hard, with shifts of 12 hours, 7 days a week, with no holidays. This lack of training affected the quality of medical care, but this was improved by the arrival from Russia, in 1880, of three certified nurses.[121] In 1881 tub baths were installed in the hospital and in 1885 another building was established with 10 beds, which operated as a ward for contagious diseases.[122]

The Russian hospital was closed at the beginning of the First World War and the staff deported as enemy citizens. The building served the Turkish army as a hospital for contagious diseases due to the epidemics which the army suffered. The Russian hospital become a British Government institution and functioned as such until 1948.[123]

Muslims Medical Activity

Turkish Municipal Hospital

The Turkish municipal hospital in Jerusalem was one of the few buildings the Turkish authorities built outside the city walls during the nineteenth century. The construction started in 1880 and was completed in 1890. The hospital, on the road to Jaffa near the local market (today 86 Jaffa Street, in the heart of Jerusalem), was two storeyed and surrounded by a thick stone wall. The hospital faced Jaffa Street and had some other small buildings on the premises for the staff and for other purposes. In 1909 a new wing for patients with contagious diseases was built by the Turkish governor.[124]

At the time of the opening, the hospital contained 32 beds and a dispensary that supplied free treatment to the farmers of the near by villages. In 1894, 890 patients of all ethnic and religion groups were hospitalized, (of which 50 died), with 1600 out-patients.[125] By 1896 the hospital had 40 beds which served both men and women (20 for each) and the staff included director, administrator, physician, surgeon, pharmacists, three nuns, seven male nurses and one female nurse.[126] The vast majority of the patients were from the poorest strata of the Holy City, and villagers, mainly Muslims. The Jews, Christians and wealthy Muslims preferred to get treatment in the modern western hospital situated nearby in Jaffa Street.

Several physicians served the municipal hospital over the years. One of the most interesting and well known physicians was Dr Photios Efklides (1864-1916), a Turk of Greek origin, who had studied medicine in Istanbul. He graduated in 1891 and was invited to practice as a physician and director of the hospital. He was also appointed as the municipal physician and received medals from the Sultan for his service in the city.[127]

In the First World War the hospital helped victims of the various epidemics that hit the city, and physicians and nurses of all religions worked together. It had sixty beds, though the sanitary conditions and medical supplies were inadequate. After the British took over the city in 1917, the building was transferred to the British governor. Beginning in 1920, the building served as the main office of the Mandate's medical department and two years later as the main medical laboratory site.[128]

Jewish Medical Activity, Institutions and Politics

The Jewish Yishuv

The Jewish community in the Land of Israel at the beginning of the nineteenth century, numbered only 6000 people, living mainly in the four cities that were considered as holy for the Jewish people: Jerusalem, Safed, Hebron and Tiberias. The majority of the Jews belonged to the *Sephardi* community living in Jerusalem, composed of fifteenth century Spanish exiles, immigrants from North Africa, and Jews who had never left the country. The *Ashkenazi* Jewish minority was divided into *Hassidim* and *Perushim* who lived mainly in Safed. In the 1880s, the mounting waves of immigration from Eastern Europe upset the balance in favor of the *Ashkenazi* community. From the 1920s onward, the *Ashkenazi* gradually began to move into Jerusalem, and in this city as in other parts of the Land of Israel, the *Ashkenazi* acquired hegemony in the Jewish community.

At the beginning of the nineteenth century, when the Jewish community was still an insignificant minority, it suffered under the strong arm of the local authorities and the Arab population, but its main affliction was extreme poverty. These conditions and the limitations placed upon the community did not allow for independent enterprise, and the Jewish *Yishuv* was dependent upon the largess of their brethren in the Diaspora. Opposition to missionary activities was one of the factors that led the Jews in the Land of Israel to rouse themselves to action on their own behalf. Even then, they were in need of the good will and funds from Jewish philanthropists and their standing in the eyes of the local authorities, in order to set up their own hospital. The first Jewish medical institutions to be built were financed by Moses Montefiore and the Rothschild family.

Later, when additional Jewish hospitals were erected, they were in need of the patronage and protection of foreign Consulates, mainly those of Austria and Germany. These hospitals will be discussed below.

The first Jewish Hospital

As a direct result of the rumours concerning the forthcoming opening of the English mission hospital in Jerusalem in early 1842, Dr Ludwig Philippson (1811-1889), a reform-minded Rabbi in Magdeburg and the editor of the German Jewish journal *Allgemeine Zeitung des Judenthums,* launched a campaign for the establishment of a Jewish hospital in Jerusalem:

> It appears that many Jews from all over the world, particularly from Eastern Europe, travel yearly to the sacred land of our forefathers. Some of them intend to stay there for some time only, others wish to spend their last years there. But in case of diseases, they are in a helpless situation… Therefore, such a hospital, provided with several scientists of our creed, would be representative of European-Jewish culture in the Orient, and a centre from which much could be achieved for the salvation of the souls of our oriental brethren…[129]

Philippson paved the way for sophisticated fund raising, involving the naming of hospital rooms after contributors, and depositing funds in European banks and sending only the interest to Jerusalem. The German philanthropists endeavored to attract potential sponsors with both religious and practical arguments. But Orthodox representatives of the Jerusalem Jews in Amsterdam, who were in charge of fund raising for the Palestinian Jews, were not ready to cooperate with the reform-minded rabbi and his supporters.[130] Philippson's campaign aroused the interest of the British Jewish philanthropist Sir Moses Montefiore. Montefiore knew the land and its Jewish inhabitants well. He paid his first visit to the Holy Land in 1827, and was president of the Board of Deputies of British Jews, and was well received in Jerusalem's orthodox community.[131]

On January 21, 1843, Philippson wrote in his editorial (*Allgemeine Zeitung des Judenthums*), in bold characters that he had important news for the interested public: Sir Moses Montefiore had decided to send the physician, Dr Shimon Fränkel to Jerusalem, to establish himself there, and to treat the poor, gratis, including medication. Sir Moses Montefiore would pay his travel costs and salary, provide him with a fully equipped pharmacy and with surgical instruments. He also guaranteed him the protection of the English Consulate and of the Turkish Governor in Jerusalem.[132]

In 1843 Moses Montefiore sent a letter to the leaders of the Jewish community in Jerusalem, as a reaction to the plans for the establishment of the English medical station in Jerusalem. The document describes the fear of the missionary work the English had started in the city:

> And when I heard that you were touched by the missionaries and three (Jewish) people were caught in their net, I was amazed, broken hearted and I cried days and nights searching for a solution… and then I met the man I am sending to you, a religious man and a physician, Dr. Simon Fränkel… God brought him to me to be sent to Jerusalem to treat our poor Jewish sick brothers… Be happy, citizens of Jerusalem… the doctor will treat you all, supply the sick ones with medications, and never again will it be said in the Holy Land, that the Jews are going to get advice from the wizards, that seduce them to leave their religions. I gave this physician drugs and medications for everybody, paid him in advance for the next three years, so he can come and take medical care of the Jewish community in Jerusalem…[133]

Dr Shimon Fränkel, aged 34, arrived in Jerusalem on April 11, 1843. He had studied medicine in Munich, and had worked for some time as a practitioner on a Dutch ship. He was married to a Jewish Caribbean woman (a Creole), which was frowned upon by the Orthodox establishment in Jerusalem. Upon arriving, the young doctor established a dispensary for the Jews in Jerusalem, not far from the English mission hospital, and even maintained a friendly and productive relationship with his English colleagues. In a letter written by Dr Edward Macgowan dated Jerusalem May 31, 1843 he described Fränkel as a physician and a colleague:

> Dr. Fränkel, the physician sent out by Moses Montefiore, has established a dispensary, and entered upon his practice among the Jews. He is very active and attentive, and has much to do. I see him frequently, and have found him a kindly disposed

> and well-informed man. His practice however, has not relieved me of any portion of my own labours among the Jews; for the number of my patients has rather increased than fallen off especially among the Sepharadim, who are consider the most respectable Jews in Jerusalem. Last week a distinguished rabbi, who was dangerously ill with Typhus fever, and whom Dr. Fränkel was attending, requested my attendance in consultation, to which Dr. Fränkel readily assented. The case terminated fatally, but I was much pleased with the attention and interest he showed to his patient.[134]

Despite the strong opposition of the representatives of the Jerusalem orthodox establishment in Amsterdam, Ludwig Philippson refused to abandon his project. The Rothschild family in Paris pledged 100,000 Francs for the establishment of the hospital, with one condition: that a school was founded at the same time.[135] But Orthodox Jews were not satisfied with these plans, fearing that the school would foster progressive European ideas and would thus endanger the faith of their children. Even Montefiore was not spared in their mistrust of the whole project.[136] Fränkel himself encouraged Philippson in a letter of October 31, 1843, stating that, more than ever, it seemed important to establish a hospital, where his cases could be treated and followed adequately. He added that the Mission institution, where only Jews were admitted, had been responsible for the conversion of 10 Jews to the Christian faith since his arrival 9 months earlier.[137]

The first Jewish hospital was probably opened at the end of 1844. John Nicolayson, the head of the London Jews Society's mission station in Palestine, described the Jewish hospital after a visit he paid to this institution:

> The house, originally one of the best in this quarter, having being used as hospital for the Egyptian soldiers [in the 1830s], has now been put into perfect repair by the Jews, and furnished with glass windows in wooden frames, painted green, as are also the inner doors. The whole house is built round a small but neat court. On the ground floor are first, a room or two occupied by a family in charge of the house, then a kitchen and a small room, in which arrangement has

> been made for heating cold water. This room served at the same time for washing the dead. Adjoining to it is another smaller room, furnished with a moveable wooden bath, to which both hot and cold water is conveyed by pipes from the other room; there is also a bed for a person to rest on, after using the bath. At the stairs that lead to the next storey is another larger room. Round the terrace, to which these stairs are three or four good-sized rooms. Two of these were occupied, one as a ward for women, the other for men. Into the latter I entered, and found, I think, six beds, four or five of which were occupied by patients… The third and last storey, where, beside a neat little room for himself [Dr Fränkel] (as manager) and also for receiving visitors, there were two very fine good-sized rooms, ventilated on all sides, and with a fine prospect through well-framed glass windows. From this terrace he also showed me a piece of ground belonging to the house, which may be turned into a garden.[138]

Swiss physician Dr Titus Tobler, visited this hospital during the winter of 1845-1846 and gave the exact location in the Jewish quarter, rather close to the English mission hospital. Tobler stresses the strength of the building, the windows of sheet-glass, and counts four sick-rooms on the second floor, and four on the third floor. The building, which was rented from Muslims, was clean and had a total of fourteen beds for the sick. Tobler observed only four female patients hospitalized. According to the staff, the number of patients sometimes reached a dozen. Nevertheless, Tobler was subtly critical of the hospital. By describing, at the same time the British hospital in Jerusalem, he mentioned the fact that the latter was the only European hospital in Palestine.[139]

As stated above, the first Jewish hospital in Jerusalem was established as a direct reaction to the establishment of the English mission hospital. The undue haste in doing so seems to have brought about its closure after only a few years. The German founder of the Deaconess Institute in Kaiserswerth, Theodor Fliender, wrote after visiting Jerusalem in 1851: 'The Jews have erected several years ago a hospital for their brethren in the Holy City. A Jewish physician from Breslau, Dr. Fränkel, was sent there…But at the time of our visit this hospital had already vanished'.[140] Titus Tobler wrote after his third visit to Jerusalem that the hospital in which Dr Fränkel was active had vanished, but that Fränkel remained in charge of the medical dispensary of Moses Montefiore.[141]

It seems that the failure of the first Jewish hospital in Jerusalem was taken into consideration by the Jewish community leaders, when planning and erecting their new hospital. And indeed, in the second half of the 1850s, when Rothschild's hospital was established, it garnered an outstanding reputation and was considered a great success. [142]

The Montefiore's Hospital

Sir Moses Motefiore continued his efforts to establish a proper Jewish hospital to provide complete medical services to Jews, and to compete with the English mission hospital. During his 1849 visit to Palestine (the third of seven) he found that a cholera epidemic had hit the Jewish community of Jerusalem, resulting in massive attendance at the English mission. Shortly after returning to England, he consulted with medical experts, and began to plan a new medical institution. He even hired two well known English architects to design the building. The drawings resemble an English palace and included communal spaces and synagogue in addition to the hospital.[143]

At the beginning of the 1850s the situation of the Jews in Palestine deteriorated. Smallpox epidemics and famine struck Jerusalem. Hunger was widespread due to the outbreak of the Crimean war in 1853 and the lack of financial support from European Jewry. The search for funds ended in 1854 with a 60,000$ bequest from Judah Touro (1775-1854), a New Orleans Jewish businessman, to improve the conditions of the Jews in the Holy Land. Touro was familiar with Montefiore's deeds and wished that after his death, the money would be used as Montefiore advised.[144] On March 25, 1854, Montefiore informed the British Prime Minister, Viscount Henry John Palmerston (1784-1865) of his 'intention of going to the East with the object of erecting a hospital at Jerusalem… which would be greatly promoted… by the Sultan allowing Jews to purchase land'.[145] Palmerston expressed his approval of the hospital but was unsure about the possibility of land acquisitions, due to the Turkish policy towards land ownership by Europeans.[146]

On his 1855 visit to Palestine, Montefiore promoted his hospital project, both by trying to obtain the Sultan's permission for building and by convincing the Touro executors to accept the plans. He travelled first to Constantinople, where he met Sir Stratford Canning (Viscount Stratford de Redcliffe 1786-1880), the British Ambassador, who was supplied with instructions to assist Montefiore in the Ottoman capital.[147] Canning managed to get Montefiore an audience with the Sultan, who remembered him from his visit 15 years earlier. The Sultan agreed to grant his request, and was 'happy to do so for my philanthropy and humanity'.[148] It is probable that Britain's support for Turkey in the ongoing Crimean War helped the Sultan to decide to approve the Montefiore hospital project.

Montefiore purchased a plot of land of 14 acres outside the city walls, on the road to Bethlehem, a few minutes walk from the Jaffa gate, for the planned hospital. The foundation stone was laid by Montefiore himself in a ceremony held on August 15, 1855.[149] But the Montefiore hospital was never erected. The three principal reasons were firstly, that it was planned to be built outside the walls in an unsafe environment; this was severely criticized. Secondly, the Rothschild hospital (to be discussed later) was already open as a well organized and well supported medical institution. Thirdly, the Rabbis of Jerusalem preferred a residential project.

The project was aborted, even though a large amount of money had already been spent on its plans. However, Touro's fund was used for another project in the same location. *Mishhkenot Sha'ananim*, a neighbourhood for poor people, was established as the first Jewish settlement outside the city walls.[150] But the significance of Montefiore's initiatives in the field of health lies not in the success or failure of his individual projects, but rather in the reformist ideas he supported. Montefiore was most likely ahead of his time in terms of what the Jewish traditionalists would tolerate.[151]

Rothschild's Hospital
(Hôpital Israelite Mayer Rothschild)

The Crimean War (1853-1856) cut the Jewish fundraising system which was the main source of income (*Chalucka*) for the Jews in Palestine during the nineteenth century. The harsh physical conditions of the Jewish community in Jerusalem caused the French members of the Rothschild family send Albert Cohn (1814-1877) to Palestine in July 1854. Cohn's main goal was to supply immediate relief by distributing money on one hand and developing long term projects on the other. Cohn was well informed about the urgent need for proper medical care for the members of the Jewish community in Jerusalem, thanks to information from Gustav de Rothschild (1829-1911), who had been sent by the family to Jerusalem a year earlier and committed the Rothschild fund to the establishment of a hospital.[152] On his way from Palestine, Cohn managed to get an appointment with the Austrian Monarch in Vienna, asking him to furnish Austrian protectorate status to the establishments recently erected in Jerusalem, including the Rothschild hospital. Such status was given because many of the Jerusalem Jews were of Austrian origin.

The Rothschild hospital in Jerusalem was opened three month after Cohn arrived there, as an eighteen-bed medical institution named after Meyer Anschel Rothschild (1744-1812) founder of the Rothschild dynasty.[153] The hospital was directed by Dr Bernhard Neumann, a native of Warsaw who had studied in Cracow and Vienna.[154] He had been in Jerusalem since 1847 and knew the city, its Jewish community and its politics quite well.[155] He described the hospital as a large building on one hill of Mount Zion, near the southern wall of the city, with a view of the Temple Mount. It included a sunny internal garden in the middle of a square building in which were located a pharmacy, offices, synagogue, staff rooms and patient rooms. The latter were large and had high ceilings. The food was decent, and the medical supplies and other equipment were sent directly from Paris. Neumann reported to Paris (with copies to Vienna and Constantinople) every four months regarding the hospital's financial activities. On average the hospital treated 600 patients every year and supplied 30,000 prescriptions.[156] In 1857, while visiting Jerusalem, Baron Alfonse de Rothschild (1827-

1905) announced, on behalf of the Rothschild family, a family decision to grant a yearly sum of 15,000 francs for the hospital. The grant was transferred every 4 months through Josef Graf von Pizzamano (1809-1860), the Austrian Consul in Jerusalem, to secure the hospital finances forever.[157]

During its first years, the Rothschild hospital faced severe management problems and suffered from the criticism of the Jewish community in Jerusalem. At first the institution was directed by a committee of 12, but following the suggestion of Pizzamano the management was given to Dr Bernhard Neumann under the direct supervision of the Austrian Consul himself. In his letter to Anton Freiherr von Prokesch-Osten (1795-1876), the Austrian delegate in Constantinople, Pizzamano referred in general to management problems in Palestine. He wrote that in order to operate any institution in the Holy City, the number of people involved should be reduced to a minimum and that the authorities provide support, both physically to protect the facility and also to be involved in its management. Otherwise, nothing could withstand the action of the 'fanaticism, illiteracy and impulses that so strongly control this miserable city'.[158]

In 1888 the new hospital building was erected outside the city walls (on 37 Ha'Neviim St. of today). It was planned by the Jerusalem architect Alexei Franghia and contained 30 beds. Dr Isaac Schwarz, who supervised the building process, handed over responsibility for supervision to Dr Isaac Grigori D'Arbela, his brother-in-law, a native of Ukraine and a French citizen, who had studied medicine in Paris.[159] Dr D'Arbela was not trusted by the members and leaders of the Jewish community, who complained frequently. In 1893, Jerusalem's *Ashkenazi* leaders sent a letter to Karl Graf von Kwiatkowski (1837-1916), the Austrian Consul, in which they declared that they had lost trust in D'Arbela. They claimed that he rejected patients, and tried to hospitalize only sure cases. They further claimed that both the food and the treatment in the hospital were of poor quality.

Rothschild sent Elijahu Scheid (1841-1922), the supervisor of the Baron's projects in Palestine, to inspect the allegations against D'Arbela. Scheid met the Austrian Consul and took the doctor's side. He determined that the Consul was not familiar with the

Orthodox Jews and their customs. Rothschild in Paris had had enough of their constant complaints. It was a known fact in Palestine that Scheid, the uncompromising supervisor, was unpopular among the Jewish settlers. The Austrian Consul sent a letter to Baron Alfonse de Rothschild and reported on the situation in the new hospital under the director Dr D'Arbela. The Consul argued that the hospital was satisfactory, and if it had a good physician, surgeon and eye doctor it could be very beneficial for the needs of the growing Jewish community in Jerusalem. He also suggested that the director of the hospital should not be a physician, but a professional administrator under whose supervision there should be a board of five people including a physician, the Consul and three leaders of the Jewish community.[160]

But not all of the physicians received such negative criticism. Dr Benjamin Rothziegel (d. 1866), who served in the Rothschild hospital in 1863-1866 during the cholera epidemic of the summer and autumn of 1865, demonstrated extraordinary devotion. During October dozens of Jerusalem's Jews died daily, and hundreds escaped from the town (among them, the local governor).[161] Rothziegel, the Jewish director of the hospital, stayed and treated his patients. In October 26, his wife died and few days later his young baby boy died too. The epidemic ended on December 30, but Rothziegel himself died a few weeks later in February 17, 1866.[162]

Bikkur Holim Hospital

Bikkur Holim was a nursing society of the *Ashkenazi* community sect of the *Perushim.* It was established in 1837 to support and treat the sick people of the community in their own homes. No physician is mentioned as practising for that society, but its activity became intensive as a result of the influence of the English medical missionaries in the city. More money was sent from Europe and Jewish leaders in Palestine and abroad had started to discuss the need for a new, modern hospital for the Jewish community in Jerusalem.[163] The community probably felt the need to establish its own hospital after the Montefiore dispensary was shut down and Dr Fränkel had left his post, and most likely as an act of opposition to the establishment of the Rothschild hospital by the *Sephardic* community.[164]

In March 26, 1863, Johann Bernhard Graf Rechberg (1806-1899), the Austrian Foreign Minister, wrote a letter to Kaiser Franz Josef and brought the request of the Jewish community to raise money in Austria, as well as asking for the Kaiser's donation for their hospital. Enclosed with the letter, is the report of the Consul in Jerusalem to the minister, requesting assistance. The Consul wrote that there was only one Jewish hospital under Austrian protection in Jerusalem, accepting all Jews, and supplying them with medical aid. The Consul referred to the hospital that was established by the Rothschild family's investment of 250,000 francs. Regarding the Bikkur Holim of the *Perushim* community, which had purchased a small house in order to furnish it as a hospital, the Consul wrote 'They intend to enlarge it by adding a few rooms and the fund raising is for that matter. Most of these people are former Russian citizens, however they had become Austrian protetti (under protection of) ten years ago'. The minister suggested, in accordance with the Consul's report, not to support their request and the Kaiser accepted the Consul's recommendation.[165]

The house in question, bought in 1865 by the Bikkur Holim society, was the former residence of the London Jews Society missionary John Nicolayson.[166] It was located between Christ Church and the English missionary hospital, and was renovated with financial aid from Moses Montefiore. The house was redesigned as a hospital, and Frankel's furniture was donated and brought in from his dispensary. Montefiore visited the building while it was under construction in April 1866, and more than a year later, on July 22, 1867 the hospital was opened, having 12 beds.[167]

The hospital did not flourish at first and for a while did not even have a physician. Its financial difficulties were solved by fundraising among a few European Jewish communities, mainly in Germany. On January 16, 1871 (just two days before the unification of Germany and the establishing of the second Reich), following a written request from the hospital's board for German protection, Max von Philipsborn on behalf of the German Chancellor, approved the request and furnished the hospital with the protection of the German Consulate in Jerusalem.[168]

A committee that had been founded in Frankfurt sent Dr Schraga Puffeles (1843-1912), a German Jewish physician, to work in Bikkur Holim hospital. The doctor, born in Cracow and medically trained in Vienna, had to work in a provisional facility. The harsh conditions in the hospital led to its closure in 1876. Later, another local Frankfurt committee took over the control of Bikkur Holim hospital with the help of the German Consulate. The new management appointed first Dr Giuseppe Carpani, physician of the French Catholic Hospital, and then, in 1886, Dr Adalbert Einsler. The Hungarian Lutheran physician had previously practiced in other institutions in the Holy Land, such as the municipal hospital in Jerusalem (1871-1887) and the German leper hospital. In 1893 the Bikkur Holim hospital had 36 beds.[169]

As an Institution under German protection, the hospital had to provide the Consulate with a yearly detailed report. In the report for 1897 one can find the following information concerning patients in Bikkur Holim: Hospitalized: 600 Men; 557 women; 95 Children. Cured: 560 Men; 502 women; 88 Children. Died: 36 Men; 48 women; 6 Children. Released without cure: 4 Men; 7 women; 1 Children. Still Hospitalized: 24 Men; 20 women; 6 Children. The report also mentioned 2 physicians; 7 administration clerks; 12 Medical staff.[170]

In November 1905 the committee of the Bikur Holim hospital in Jerusalem (Moshe Yoel Solomon 1835-1913, Yehiel Michael Pinnes 1854-1913 and Asher Eliezer Levi) under the patronage of the German Consulate, requested once more the permission of the Austrian Consul to conduct fundraising in the Austrian kingdom for the relief of the hospital. In their letter to the Home Office in Vienna, the committee members described the financial difficulties of the hospital and the medical needs of the Jewish community in Jerusalem. They could not cover the growing expenses and therefore asked permission to raise funds within the Jewish community in Austria. Their main argument was that the Austro-Hungarian Jewish community benefited much from this institution. They most likely referred to the Rothschild hospital under Austrian protection that was not fulfilling the medical needs of the Austrian Jews in Jerusalem. Heinrich Jehlitschka, the Acting Consul in Jerusalem added some remarks to his covering letter, stating that the hospital was one of the best managed senior Jewish medical institutions in the city, serving the growing Jewish community, mainly the poor. The Consul mentioned (probably what the Jewish committee wished to mention as well but chose not to) that the Rothschild hospital, the only Jewish hospital, which was under Austrian protection, could not accept all the members of the Austrian-Hungarian community. The Consul supported the request and it was almost certainly approved.[171]

Dr Einsler proved himself a good choice and under his management the hospital was successful. In May 1910, after the premises became too small for its activity, a cornerstone for a new building was laid outside the walls of the old city. It was located between the new German Consulate and the hospital of the German Deaconesses of Kaiserswerth (on the corner of Ha'Neviim and Strauss St. of today). Building was interrupted by the outbreak of the First World War. Only in April 1925, was the new Bikkur Holim hospital inaugurated. It still functions as a hospital today.

Shaare Zedek Hospital

Attempts to establish another Jewish hospital in Jerusalem commenced in 1884 by forming a Jewish committee in Germany which bought the old residence of the German Consulate in Jerusalem. Negotiations were conducted between Dr Mayer Lehmann, the head of the Jewish committee for establishing the new hospital, Julius Reitz, the German Consul, Joseph Maria von Radowitz (1839-1912), the German Ambassador in Constantinople and Mehmed Rauf Pasha, the Ottoman Governor of Jerusalem. The negotiations ended with a Turkish refusal, mainly because the building was in the Muslim Quarter of the city, and the Arab neighbours objected to having a hospital at their back door. The official argument by the Governor was that an inspection committee of physicians determined that the hospital would not be safe for the health of the nearby residents. After the German Consul appealed against the physicians' report by bringing in another professional opinion, the Governor came up with another argument. He declared that in an intermixed city, one community can not build its institutions in another community's dwelling quarter. The project was denied.[172]

The Jewish committee for establishing the new hospital renewed its effort by sending Dr Moritz (Moshe) Wallach (1866-1957), an Orthodox Jew from Cologne, to Jerusalem in 1891. He graduated in medicine in 1889 as a general practitioner in gynaecology, ophthalmology, dentistry and paediatrics. After practising as a private physician, he was hired as the physician of the Bikkur Holim hospital and played a major role in obtaining land and establishing the Shaare Zedek hospital.[173]

From the start, Dr Wallach faced the authorities' refusal of his attempt to purchase the land necessary for the hospital. At that time, two years after the massive acquisition of land by the new Jewish immigrants, the Ottoman Empire had restricted that option for non-Muslims in Palestine. As a physician of the Bikkur Holim hospital under German protection and as a German patriot, Wallach looked for assistance from Fürst Hugo von Radolin (1841-1917), the German Ambassador in Constantinople. Radolin encouraged Paul von Tischendorf (1847-1914), the German Consul in Jerusalem, to assist Wallach since Germany was in favour of that project.[174] The negotiations were conducted for more than two years and, eventually in October 1895, the firman for the registration of the land under Jewish owners was given, together with permission to build the hospital.

In 1894, during the negotiations, Wallach purchased a piece of land, outside the walls of the old city, near the Shaare Zedek settlement, from Johannes Frutiger (1836-1899) the Swiss owner of the largest private bank in Jerusalem.[175] The plans for the new building were drawn up by Jerusalem German architects Conrad Schick and Theodor Sandel. Construction started in 1897 and provided work for members of the Jewish community for more than five years.[176]

The Shaare Zedek hospital was inaugurated on January 27, 1902 (on 161 Jaffa St. of today), as one of the largest premises in Jerusalem, 80 metres long and 30 metres wide. The two storey building contained 80 beds and a modern, well equipped operating theatre. The first floor was used for clinics, pharmacy, offices, physicians' rooms and kitchen. The second floor accommodated the in-patient rooms in different departments for men, women and children. The cellar was used as storage room for the food, drugs and other medical supplies. The building was surrounded by a large garden and a protective stone wall. Two small buildings on the ground were used to accommodate patients with contagious diseases, as well as premises for nurses.[177]

Several months after the opening of the hospital, Dr Wallach sent a detailed report to Edmund Schmidt (1855-1916), the German Consul in Jerusalem. He stated that the main building, the two minor buildings for isolation against contagious diseases, the laundry facilities and the disinfection installation were all hygienically acceptable. The hospital was designated to treat the poor Jews of Jerusalem free of charge but at the time (August 1902) only the women's and children's department were fully operational. The staff included a physician and administrator, 6 nurses and 21 other employees. The clinic was open everyday but Saturday, for every patient, regardless of religion, free of charge. About 100 patients with eye diseases, internal diseases and surgical needs visited the clinic every day.[178]

Misgav Ladach Hospital

When the Rothschild hospital was founded in 1854 in the building belonging to the *Sephardi* community of Jerusalem, it was agreed that if one day the hospital moved to another location, the old building would be returned to the *Sephardi* community. Accordingly, in 1888, when new premises were built for the Rothschild hospital outside the city walls, the building in the old city was delivered to the Misgav Ladach Society. This Society had been founded in 1879 by wealthy Jews from Salonika. It had 300 members in its first year and in its third year as many as 1,300 members. It was operated as a 'sick fund', or a type of health insurance, the first among the Jewish community in the Holy Land. The members of the society were entitled to receive medical care and medicines for a monthly membership. This arrangement kept the society as an independent institution not under the leaders of the *Sephardi* community who controlled the distribution of charity funds to the Jewish population. At first, the society opened and operated a pharmacy, in which a few Jewish pharmacists practiced over the years. The last pharmacist was Moshe Rubowitch who had trained in the Rothschild hospital, and who later directed the pharmacy of the

Misgav Ladach hospital. Rububitch also deputised for the physicians when they were on leave. Later, the society hired its own physician, one of the best in Jerusalem at this time, Dr Kalermo Mazaraky of Greek Christian origin. Dr Mazaraky overcharged his uninsured patients but thanks to a special arrangement, the members of the Misgav Ladach Society paid only a quarter of this fee.[179]

The Misgav Ladach society intended to operate its own hospital, without the protection of any foreign Consulate. Accordingly, in 1889 the society inaugurated a hospital in its building, despite the fact that the directors and administrators of the Rothschild hospital convinced the Turkish authorities that the building was no longer suitable to serve as a hospital. Soon it become the only hospital within the walls of the old city, and it therefore gained a special importance.[180] The planned institution was described in detail in the society literature:

> the upper storey will consist of seven big rooms for the patients, and an operating theatre. The lower storey will be occupied by a synagogue, a library, a Yeshiva, pharmacy, the society house, two dispensaries, kitchen, dining room, Mikve (ritual bath), laundry room and a separate room for the contagious diseased. The garden will be a place for walking for the sick.[181]

Although the Misgav Ladach hospital was founded by the *Sephardi* community in Jerusalem, it welcomed patients from all ethnic groups. For example, in 1896, the dispensary treated 2616 *Sephardi* Jews, 2480 *Ashkenazi* and 91 Muslims. Between 1879 and 1896 (seventeen years) the hospital had 2817 inpatients, out of which 1490 were men and 1327 women. 178 patients died in the hospital during this period and 65,000 outpatients were treated. The hospital supplied altogether 40,430 free prescriptions.[182] In 1890 the hospital had 67 beds. In 1898 the building of a new ward was completed and in the same year a wealthy Jew from Bukhara donated five beds and named them after Emil Zola (1840-1902) for his efforts to clear the allegation against Alfred Dreyfus (1859-1935), the Jewish French officer who had been accused of betraying his nation four years before. In 1907-1908 the hospital had 50 beds and three pharmacists and two physicians worked there, Dr Nikafury Mazaraky (brother of K. Mazaraky) and Dr Avraham Aboujedid (1875-1930) the first Palestine-born Jewish physician. Aboujedid, a French citizen, studied medicine in Istanbul and was hired by Dr K. Mazaraky as his assistant.[183]

In 1914 the budget could not be balanced and some of the employees left the hospital due to the outbreak of the First World War that forced subjects of the Allies to leave Palestine. The hospital survived the first two years of the War with donations from the USA government and other sources. The physicians continued to visit the patients and operate the dispensaries. In 1916 a typhus epidemic hit the city and the Turkish authorities evacuated the hospital and used it for the typhus victims; this time the number of Jewish patients was less than a half. Near the end of the war the building was taken over by the Ottoman authorities and the Turkish soldiers destroyed it almost completely. After the war, in 1918, the leaders of the Misgav Ladach Society and the management of the institution decided to reopen the hospital. However, this was not an easy task. The society declined offers of support from outsiders, if they had to change their location or reopen as a small hospital. The leaders struggled to obtain financial aid from all over the world, with almost no success. Nevertheless, many well known physicians of the Jewish community in Jerusalem practised in this institution, mainly during the 1930s and 1940s.[184]

Misgav Ladach hospital was the last functioning hospital in the old city of Jerusalem after the other medical institutions had relocated in new buildings outside the city walls, and was the first hospital to be completely destroyed after the Jordanian army overran the Jewish Quarter in 1948. A new temporary Misgav Ladach Hospital was established, a short time later in 1948, in the new city of Jerusalem and later a permanent hospital was built on 27 Ha'Melech Hizkia St. of today).[185]

POSTSCRIPT

Never in modern history have such concentrated efforts been made to establish medical institutions and to care for the health and welfare of so small a population in such a narrow geographical space as in the Land of Israel. Never have so many nations, so many emissaries of so many religious institutions and missionary societies, so many heads of communities and so many individual philanthropists invested such tremendous financial resources as were invested in establishing hospitals in the Holy Land during the nineteenth century. Never have the inhabitants of this strip of land experienced such a radical change in the way and expectancy of life they enjoyed through medical institutions that were provided with the most highly advanced equipment then in existence. Within the short period of only 70 years, from the construction of the first hospital in 1844 until the eve of the First World War in 1914, in the little city of Jerusalem (with a population of only 70,000 inhabitants), there stood some 15 hospitals with hundreds of beds for patients.

This process, which helped to transform the Land of Israel from medieval darkness to modern times, was began by a modest English Mission Society trying to spread the gospel among the Jews of Palestine in order to hasten the days of redemption. The most efficient means for religious conversion during the nineteenth century was the medical mission, and thus, by the 1820s, the London Jews Society had sent its first physician-missionary to the Holy Land. This initiative led to the establishment of the first Western-style hospital in the Holy Land and, indirectly, to the establishment of many other medical institutions.

British engagement in missionary work among the Jews, and the emphasis given to doing so through medical practices, set in motion a process that transformed the face of the Land of Israel. The meteoric rise of medicine in the Holy Land is due first and foremost to the competition that developed among the players in this field. Moreover, the competition to provide medical services was one 'front' in the battle among European competitors for control of this region. It was the wretched state of health among the Jews of Jerusalem that instigated the process by which modern missionary medicine established itself in the Land of Israel.

Despite these distressing health conditions, the leaders of the Jewish community were mainly engaged in the difficulties of communal survival, in the raising of funds for subsistence and in its distribution among their flock. Before the arrival of the British, no effort was made to raise funds for the founding of hospitals. However, when the gates of the first English hospital opened in 1844, the Jewish community leaders feared the missionary component of the hospitals and attempted to prevent their people from using the services of the medical institution, and at the same time set up their own competing medical institution.

As if the hostile competition between the Jewish community and the English mission was not enough, internal rivalry over medical issues began among members within the Jewish community. A struggle developed between ultra-orthodox and more liberal Jews over the character of the hospitals and institutions associated with them. Disputes arose between *Ashkenazim* and *Sephardim* that were mainly due to attempts to obtain hegemony within the Jewish community. These struggles reflected a need to gain the support of European Jewish philanthropists, and furtive competition was created between the French house of Rothschild with its *Ashkenazi* orientation and Moses Montefiore, the Englishman of Italian origins with his *Sephardi* orientation. It even seemed as though their national affiliations, one from Catholic France and the other from Protestant England were an inherent part of the undercurrent of competition between the medical institutions they had established. Throughout that century, Jewish communities set up additional hospitals in Jerusalem, and because of the hostile character of the Ottoman regime, they needed the protection of other European powers. Germany and Austria were quick to offer their protection to the medical institutions set up by the Jews of Jerusalem who held European nationality, and this fact added a further dimension to the existing competition.

Yet is seems that the strongest competition in the medical field developed among the powers as part of their attempts to win priority status in the Holy Land and the fear of being displaced by other European rivals. This competition was motivated by the political and economic issues in the framework of 'The Eastern Question' that occupied Europe during most of the nineteenth century. The main issue was: Who among the powers would gain portions of the disintegrating Ottoman Empire? Among other interests of concern was the desire of Russia to enable the masses of Russian pilgrims to visit the Holy Land freely; to protect the Arab Orthodox community that constituted the majority of Christians in the Land of Israel; and to take control over the holy places. The foremost concern of the British was to ensure a safe route to the East and to India that passed close by the Land of Israel, and religious concern with the Jewish community in the country in relation to the idea of the 'Restoration of the Jews'. France wanted to preserve its traditional status as the protector of Christianity in the Land of Israel and the links between the Catholic Church under its protection and the sacred sites. This competition was evident in many areas, including the creation of 'national' hospitals in Palestine. The results of this competition led, as stated before, to essential changes in the quality and expectancy of life for the inhabitants of the country – Jews, Muslims, and Christians. The large numbers of hospital beds for patients in the many hospitals and the masses of people that constantly streamed through them, attracted skilled foreign and Jewish physicians from Europe. The medical quality that they generated increased during the years of the British Mandate in Palestine and laid the foundations for the achievements that placed the State of Israel at the forefront of research and as one of the most important medical centres in the world.

However, the picture of medical realities portrayed here, in which the British missionaries played a central role, and in which other factors contributed towards medical advancement, would not be complete without one reservation. The medical institutions fulfilled their task of curing the sick among the local population with great success, but they did not succeed in changing the bad sanitary conditions and the low standards of cleanliness among the inhabitants of the country during the nineteenth century. The missionaries and all those engaged in medical activities did their best to educate the public and to change its habits, but the local Ottoman regime was indifferent, even obstructing their work and preventing them from carrying out the desired changes. In time, the Governor of Jerusalem was also drawn into the competition and established a municipal hospital, but this occurred only towards the end of the nineteenth century, about fifty years after the first Western-style hospital was established. Only the change in the existing regime by British rule in 1918 made it possible to complete the revolution.

The best, most meticulous description of the sanitary conditions in Jerusalem at the end of the period under discussion was contained in a report prepared by Percy d'Erf Wheeler, Medical Superintendent of the English Mission Hospital and Ernest Masterman, of the Department of Public Health in Jerusalem. The report was sent to John Dickson (1846-1906), British Consul in Jerusalem:[1]

> The present state of affairs is a standing danger to British residents and visitors, but with the plague so near at hand, to leave things as they are is to invite a disaster. Jerusalem is extraordinarily well furnished with private hospitals supported by various foreign Societies & there are many medical men of all nations, but… nothing so far is being done or can by private individuals be done, to improve a condition of things which… is a disgrace to civilization… Piles of vegetable & animal substances in a rotting condition… are left there for days & often even months. Secondly, in all but the main streets & especially under archways (where foul air can specifically accumulate) it is the custom for the people to answer the calls of nature whenever convenient to themselves… The above mentioned nuisances lay the inhabitants & visitors of this city open to constant attacks of

> Malaria, Dysentery, Diarrhoea & Enteric Fever, but they also directly & indirectly open the road for epidemics of a serious nature… Our hands, as private medical men, are powerless to strike at the roots of the evil… there is not a single hospital bed in Jerusalem open to the poor for any infectious disease.

Thus the main factor that affected the health of the inhabitants of the Land of Israel even at the end of the period in question after the establishment of so many Western-style hospitals, was the pernicious sanitary conditions that remained unchanged. Infectious diseases were and continued to be the main obstacle in improving the life expectancy of the inhabitants. This fact raises another issue that has to remain unresolved in the framework of this study. Among the many hospitals that were established by the European powers in the wake of the English Mission, were those established, for the first time in the Land of Israel, in response to a particular medical need. An English hospital was built for eye diseases and a German hospital for lepers. This fact raises the question: Why were special medical institutions built for these particular purposes and how is it that not a single medical institution was built, for example, to offer special treatment for the infectious diseases that were many times more widespread? In most of the London Jews Society hospitals it appears that treatment was given for similar needs. Cataract operations and treatment for the restoration of eyesight were extensively carried out. Pharmacies and outpatient clinics of the Society treated most of the orthopaedic cases for the restoration of motor ability. Might there have been some hidden intent in selecting these areas for medical specialization? Not a single document has been found as evidence of this, and any such question probably will remain unanswered. Despite realistic doubts, it could be suggested that a hint regarding this issue may be contained in the account of an English priest who had been invited to visit the pharmacy of the English Mission Hospital in Jerusalem, published by the London Jews Society in a modest booklet certainly intended for gaining adherents among Christian believers:

> It was the close of a ten days' tour round about Jerusalem, and we were standing on the steps of the splendid hospital belonging to the London Jews' Society… As agreed we set

out the following morning for our inspection… The doctor [Percy d'Erf Wheeler] was sitting down at his desk to receive the first patient… The patient was a young man who limped. The doctor pointed him to a stool by his side, and said some kindly words. He spoke in Arabic, which we did not understand, but the interpretation was given to us in an answering smile of the young Jews' face. At another word the patient stretched out his leg, and the doctor unwound a bandage. There was approval on the medical face... 'Yes', he said, 'He'll do'… 'I thought he would have lost his leg. He'll do now'…

A poor woman… came through, sat down on the stool, and showed the doctor her baby. It was about eighteen months old, blind! The poor little creature lay on the mother lap quite still, its eyelids closed – just a pathetic bit of human weakness. The woman said nothing, but looked at the doctor with an appeal in her face that was more eloquent than many words. He bent towards the mother, and there was a fine tenderness in his look. He gently touched the closed eyelids, and bade her be of good cheer. The baby should be made quite well, and would be able to see... The woman seized his hand, kissed it, and rose and went out, her face radiant. As she wrapped her covering round the baby and looked down on the little face she smiled. It was a smile that almost brought tears to our eyes… It seemed a repetition of what is to be read in the pages of our Gospel…

We went out… Said one of the party: 'we have seen a sight in old Jerusalem that we shall not forget. Isn't it all like a bit of the Acts of the Apostles? Here in the very city where the Lord taught and suffered is His work still going on. We have seen Him this morning. His hands are working in that little room. His love and power manifest themselves through that doctor. As of old so to-day, the Lord is present to heal.[2]

APPENDIXES

Appendix 1 - List of Household Furniture in the English mission hospital in Jerusalem

The list below was found in the Journal written by the head of the English mission hospital in Jerusalem, dated December 29, 1860, for the purpose of inventory at the beginning of Dr Thomas Chaplin's post. The document gives us a unique opportunity to learn in detail about one aspect of the physical conditions, e.g. the instruments that had been used by practitioners as well as by the patients in the hospital. It includes furniture, as well as implements that had been used in the kitchen and the dining rooms and more importantly, the medical equipment.

By exploring the list one can say that the vast majority of the household, furniture, domestic and surgical tools were brought from England. A closer look at the surgical instruments shows us that they were very modern at that time and were similar to those used in England and the colonies at that time.

Special attention should be paid to the tools that were used to perform 'old fashioned' procedures such as a 'Porcelain Bleeding Basin' and a 'Portable cupping case', the diagnostic tools such as: 'Old Stethoscopes and 1 Flexible ditto'. Interesting tools and apparatus are: 'Old Injection apparatus' and 'Tin Case of 12 Vaccine Bottles. Bottles nearly all broken'. Special apparatus for the beginning and cessation of life are: a 'Leather Case of Midwifery Instruments', and a 'Post Mortem Case – Mahogany'.

Evidence uf early use of very modern medical procedures can be found in the existence of: 'Apparatus for Inhaling (Chloroform)' that was used for anesthesia while operating, and the set of tools for various operational procedures: 'Amputation and operations on the Eye, Teeth and Ear – For Fistula Lackeymales, stone in the Bladder, also a complete Set of Catheters, Sounds and Bougies Scalpels, Specula, Dislocation Apparatus etc.'

Evidence perhaps of the earliest use of complementary medicine in the Holy Land comes from the existence of: a 'Small Case Homeopathic Medicinal going to England by Capt. Layard'.

Of special interest were the modern electric devices: 'Mahogany Case cont. Electro-Magnetic Apparatus – Glass Case', and 'Case cont. large Electrical Machine'.

List of Household Furniture left for the use of the physician, Jerusalem December 29, 1860[3]

1 large iron Bedstead, with Mattress. Bolster and 2 pillows
1 Small 3 ft. Camp-bed-stead in case complete with 2 Mattresses and Bolster and Pillow
2 Teak-wood side table
1 Oak-wood Dinning Table with 3 Space-leaves of fir, oak edged
1 Sofa-table with Flaps and 2 Drawers (1 key)
1 small Mahogany round Table
1 Mahogany side board with 4 drawers – 1 plate chest and 1 back-drawer with 3 keys
1 Mahogany Sofa covered with red Damask and 2 pillows
1 Teak wood Sofa cotton back hided with mattresses and two pillows…
1 Beechwood folding Easy Chair
2 Arm & 18 Drawing Room Chairs with rail at back…
1 Iron reclining Chair, with rest for legs
1 Large Turkey Carpet 15 x 10 ft.
4 Painted Garden Stool (Chair)
1 Night Chair
1 Swing Sofa Lamp with pulleys…
1 Garden Flower Stand painted green
1 … Bread Pan
2 Stoves with fire irons & fittings complete
1 Oak Wood Chest of Drawers with key
1 Round table
1 Oblong Breakfast Table
9 Bed Room Chairs …bottomed, old & rickety, all broken to pieces
1 Cane-bottomed Arm Chair
1 Cane-bottomed without Arms

1 Wash-hand stand – 2 Basin + 1 Jug cracked – 2 sets of Soap & Brush and imperfect dishes
1 Duping table
1 Toilet – Glass-Mahogany-complete
1 Dual Towel Horse
1 Damask Table Cover, very old, in Library
1 Bread Basket
5 Casseroles or Saucepans… useless
3 Iron Sauce Pans – enamelled
2 Frying Pans
1 Pudding Dish metal…
1 Iron Tea Kettle
1 Large coffee boiler
1 Chopper
1 Tin Watering Pot – old and gone
3 Iron Fire Stand
1 Hand Bell
2 Lanterns – worn out
1 Garden Spade – new…
1 Brass Lamp
1 pair Balance Scales with 3 iron Weights- borrowed by S. Weissmann
9 Bone Egg or Salt Spoons
1 Etna – (Spirit)
2 Salt… glass
3 Table Cloths - worn out
4 Table Napkins - worn out
5 Towels - worn out
2 pair sheets - worn out
1 white Bed Quilt - worn out
1 Red & White Coverlet - worn out
Foot Vallance for large Bed & Mosquito Curtain
4 Toilet Covers
11 Ivory – handled – Table knives – old
8 do " Dessert "
5 do " Forks "
1 Carving Knife & Fork –
1 Brass Funnel
1 Strong Box tin-lines… painted black

Effects in Dispensary Dec.28th.1860

1 Writing Desk, in recess with lock & key. -
1 Counter with Drawers
2 pairs large brass Scales with weights
2 " small "
1 Twin Roller
1 Table Scales & weights
1 Hanging Solar Oil Lamp
2 Buckets
1 Spirit Lamp
8 Funnels…
5 Pestles
2 Tincture… – 1 Piston deficient
2 Large Water Jugs – one handle off
2 Small " 1 cracked
1 Plaster Machine
2 Pill machines
1 Powder Mill – cylinder worn out

2 Porcelain Slabs – 4
1 Large Still
1 Small "
1 Foot Tub
1 Iron Bucket & Rope – now a chain
2 Water Casks – old also 2 new ones
188 Small Drawers & 11 small closets
1 Large… Cabinet with Shelves
20 Large Black Bottles for Medicines
1 Cork Presser with Knife (Knife broken)
35 Infusion Pots with Covers (12 blue, quite new)
30 Shelves
15 Glass Measures (3 broken)
16 Spatula with 1 wooden one
1 Box chemical…
1 Box containing chemical
Apparatus with pneumatic Sroughike
1 Medical Chest (empty one new and good, two old)
2 Sieves
1 Filtering Machine
1 Large Stone Spirit Jar
A number of Glass tubes and rods
1 Large Iron Mortar…
1 Tin Basin
15 Ointment Pots
35 Extracts "
39 Narrow Mouthed, white stoppered Bottles – labels – quarters
39 Wide "
45 Narrow " pints
27 Wide "
20 Blue Syrup Bottles -
" quarters
52 White narrow mouth Stopper Bottles, not all labeled, 4 to 8 ozs
45 " Sundry Green Glass bottles of Sizes
8 Old Mesh bottomed (hair)…
1 Brass Funnel candle stick
1 Iron Stove with Piping complete in upper room over Dispensary
5 Wooden Chairs – two without backs
5 Pewter measures – pint & half pint 1 ladder

Effects in Room occupied by Mr. Wiseman

1 Table
1 Wash Stand with Basin and Jug
1 High Desk and Stool – sent to Hospital out-patient room.
Iron Bedstead with… Mattress – returned to Hospital
4 Blankets – one old – worn out long ago
1 Iron Stove – old
3 Chairs – old
1 Brass Coffee Pot
1 Brass kettle

Surgical Instruments and Sundry Apparatus

1 Portable Iron Case, containing Trephining & Amputating Instruments
1 Porcelain Bleeding Basin
1 Leather Case of Midwifery Instruments old
1 Leather Case of Midwifery Instruments new
1 Portable cupping case
1 case cont. 3 Uterine Specula (Glass)
2 Small cases cont. 2 white bulac
1 Hydrocele Case – imperfect
1 Case Flumier (?) Specula
1 Post Mortem Case Mahogany
1 Bivalve Speculum
1 Brass Candle Lamp, with Speculum…
1 Tin Case of 12 Vaccine Bottles. Bottles nearly all broken.
2 Old Stethoscopes and 1 Flexible ditto
1 Apparatus for Inhaling (Chloroform)
1 pair Small Scales – weights sent to Dispensary
6 Male Syringes. Worn out
1 Breast Pump
1 Small Case Homeopathic Medicinal - going to England by Capt. Layard
1 Old Injection apparatus
1 Stand cont. 8 Spuel Lamps with 2 Urinconnector
A lot of Splints, Bandages, syringes etc.
Hernia Trusses
1 India Rubber Post mortem Injector Apparatus
2 Sets of Waterproof dissecting Aprons and Sleeves
1 Mahogany Case cont. Electro-Magnetic Apparatus – Glass Case
1 Case cont. large Electrical Machine
1 Case cont .Chemical Apparatus
1 Mahogany Cabinet with Drawers by Weiss – containing Instruments for Amputation and operations on the Eye, Teeth and Ear – For Fistula Lachrymalis, stone in the Bladder, also a complete Set of Catheters, Sounds and Bougies Scalpel, Specula, Dislocation Apparatus etc.
1 Shower Bath…
1 Vapour Bath apparatus in case
1 Newman's Mountain Barometer
1 Ivory double-tubed Thermometer – broken
1 Connenson Thermometer – now broken by wind

Men's Large Ward

8 Iron Bedsteads with mattresses, Pillows etc.

8 Eight Tables with Drawers
1 Deal Table with Drawers
8 Windsor Chairs
3 Lockers with padlocks and keys
2 Copper Dishes
1 Pewter bleeding Basin
3 Iron Cradles for Surgical Cases
1 Basin with Jug

Small Accident Ward

2 Iron Bedstead with bedding complete
2 Small Night Tables
2 Windsor Chairs
1 Iron Washing Stand

Women's Large Ward

10 Iron Bedstead with bedding complete
7 Night Tables
1 Old Iron Stove – incl. piping
1 Iron Wash-hand Stead with Basin
1 Large Brass Basin
1 Copper Tray for burning Charcoal
1 Pewter Bleeding Basin
1 Brass Pestle and Mortar

Small Women's Ward.

4 Iron Bedsteads with bedding complete
4 Night Tables
1 Round painted Deal Table
1 Iron Wash-hand Stand with Basin
3 Windsor Chairs, two are Rush-bottomed
1 Copper Caldron
1 Large Copper Basin
1 Box for Sundries

Matron's Rooms

6 Rush-bottomed … Chairs - new
1 Mahogany Folding Table
1 Setter & Mattress
1 Painted …Clothes Press
1 " square Table with Drawers
1 Stove with piping – Boiler and Tap complete
1 Painted chest of drawers
1 Wash Hand Table, Basin and Jug
1 Water Can
1 Box for Sundries
1 Round painted Deal Table

Steward's Bed Room – upstairs

1 Mahogany folding Table
1 Dressing Table
1 Painted Wash hand Stand
1 Night Table
3 painted rush-bottomed chairs
1 Stove with piping
1 Easy Chair

Children's Rooms – downstairs

1 Painted Round Table
1 Chest of Drawers – 5 Drawers

1 Iron Bed with Mattress & 2 pillows & Blankets from Mr. Calman
5 Painted Rush bottomed Chairs – old
1 " Wash Hand Stand
1 Tin Water Can
1 Mattress, 4 Sheets, 4 Pillows

Porter's Room

1 ...Table (Dressing)
1 Windsor Chair

Recess in Accident Ward

1 Winnowing Machine – sold by Capt. Layard and family
2 Tin Baths – full sized - one sold
1 Table for rubbing Paint
1 Pair Spare Iron Trestles for Bed in Doctor's House
1 Large patent Weighting Machine with 10 weights
4 spare Iron Bed stead with mattresses and pillows
5 do. Night Table
3 old Night Stools
1 Iron Wire Guard for Window
1 Saw
1 Axe
1 Carpenter's Hone

The Hall

1 Mahogany Dining Table
1 Deal writing Table
1 Setter with Mattress and covering
8 Rush-bottomed Chairs
1 Stove with piping
2 Large Clothes Presser
2 Small " "
3 Tea Trays
3 Water Bottles
6 Tumblers
8 Metal Tea Spoons
3 do. Table do,
5 Brass " "
10 Black handled Knives
2 Metal Teapots – old
4 Cups and Saucers...
3 Dishes
1 Salt Cellar
1 Tea Caddy
2 Brass Saucepans
6 Basins
4 Stone Jars
1 Graduated Glass Measure – broken
1 Wedgwood Mortar and Pestle
1 Brass Drinking Cup – new
2 Old Window Curtains
3 Floor Mats
1 Tin Canister for Tea
1 Portrait in Oil of Dr. Macgowan
Human Skull and Bones
3 Old Table Clothes (Covers)

Patient Waiting Room

Mattress & 3 Blankets in Locker for Porter
2 Benches

Consulting Room

1 Round... Table
1 Iron Wash-hand Stand and Basin

5 Chairs – rush-bottomed
1 Bench
1 Iron Bedstead, Mattress and Pillows
1 Floor Mat

Baker's Room

1 New Stool and pipe
2 Curtains for Windows

Grain and Oil Store

5 Large Deal Chests for Wheat
2 Small "
7 Large… Jars for Oil
3 Large Southern Buckets – 1 new

Store Room near Kitchen

8 Cases with Locks for Sugar, Coffee and tea
1 Wooden Grain Measure

Kitchen and Bakery

8 Copper Saucepans of diff[erent] sizes – 3 with covers
2 Copper Trays
1 do, Mortar and Pestle
5 Brass Dishes
2 do Jugs
2 Tin "
6 Iron Milk Saucepans – one with cover
3 do, " "
1 Iron pan for roasting Coffee…
2 Iron Strainers
4 " Stands or Tripods and 2 large ones
1 pair of Scales for Bread - with weights
1 " " " with brass pans - with weights
3 Iron Tea Trays – old
3 Shovels for Fire and Oven – 1 wood – 1 iron rake
1 Small Pepper Mill
Coffee Boiler – 3 large boilers
2 Barrels for Water…
3 Wooden Wash Tubs
1 Large… Table
1 pair Fire Tongs
2 Meat Chopper and Block
1 Table – fixed to wall under Shed in court
1 Wooden Trough for Kneading
1 Large Coffee Kettle
1 Tin Coffee Pots
24 " Plates – 3 tin frying pans
3 Lamps (Pump)
9 Lanterns
12 Spittoons for Patients

Sundries

1 Canvas Covering for Terrace
1 Stretcher
2 Large Ladders
1 Folding Steps
1 Large Coffee Mill
1 Mangle
1 Ironing Table
1 Iron Crow Bar
1 Iron Shovel
1 Pick Axe
1 Hoe

Appendix 2 - The first pages of Dr. Macgowan's private journal

Dr Edward Macgowan - a physician in Exeter, joined the ranks of the London Jews Society for the purpose of establishing the first modern hospital in the Holy Land - arrived in the city of Jerusalem on January 21, 1842. Macgowan started practising medicine among the Jews of Jerusalem right away, and after several months he began recording his personal impressions in a hand-written Journal. The following appendix presents the first pages of the journal from May 31, 1842. Macgowan wrote throughout the years he spent as head of the medical mission in Jerusalem until his death in 1860. His successors, Dr Thomas Chaplin and Dr Percy d'Erf Wheeler continued writing, in a briefer and more official manner, in the same journal until December 31, 1899.

In this part of the Journal, Macgowan reported his initial impressions of the awkward and dangerous work in his first weeks in Jerusalem. Among other issues, he wrote, more than 2 years before he established the hospital, about the first technical arrangements in the dispensary and the accommodation of the missionaries. He described his daily routine in the dispensary and the lack of medical education and hygiene among the Jews in the Holy City. He also portrayed the main diseases of which the people of Jerusalem suffered from, e.g. fevers, typhus, dysentery and eye diseases, including trachoma, on which, according to the Journal, he could not operate at that early stage. The Journal recounts of first hand the medical condition of Jerusalem and its inhabitants, and the first interaction between the Jews and the English medical missionaries.

This primary source, written during the long evenings after a day of work, presents Macgowan's processing of the daily events and experiences, the medical as well as the human aspects of practising. The personal way in which the Journal was written expresses the excitement and depressions, highlights and frustration that the first Western practitioner in the Holy Land had experienced.[4]

May 31, 1842, JOURNAL

Since my first report which was forwarded from Jerusalem in the month of March last, I have been engaged in carrying into execution the plan which I had then commended for the establishment of the dispensary. The surgery and drugs have been removed from their former inconvenient situation into a small adjoining house which is better adapted for the purpose, and which contains also the accommodation of bedroom and sitting room for W. Bergheim. The structure of the Lingery [sic.] which I purchased in London had been very neatly put up in these premises by our German carpenter, quite in the English style. They make a very respectable appearance and have given no little surprise and satisfaction to the English travellers who have paid us a visit. This arrangement affords more room in the house previously appropriated for that purpose and which is my present residence. I had hoped that it would have afforded sufficient accommodation for me; but now [that] all our surgical and medical apparatus has arrived, in addition to my own library, I find that it is much too small to contain the whole. The arrangement therefore which I have proposed to the Bishop, which he has approved of, is that I should provide a more suitable dwelling for myself and leave the whole of the present premises to be appropriated to the Dispensary and for a lodging for the dispenser. They are by no means too large for that purpose, especially as it is Mr. Bergheim's intention to become a family man, of which circumstance he has given the Bishop and myself a written communication. I take this opportunity of conveying to the Committee my satisfaction with Mr. Bergheim both on account of his general good conduct as of great attention to the duties of his situation. He is very desirous of pursuing his medical studies but at present his time is so fully engaged in his own department that it is not possible for him to find leisure to do so. A considerable part of his time is taken up with officiating as interpreter for myself with the patient who attends the Dispensary during which he is necessarily prevented from dispensing the medicines which have been prescribed. In consequence of this double occupation he is generally engaged until a late hour in the evening, and precluded from taking exercise in the open air without the wall of the city, which is very undesirable.

It has occurred to me to remedy this inconvenience by engaging for the present, an Interpreter, which will release Bergheim from that duty and leave him more time for his other occupations. I have found a respectable and intelligent Jew. A married man, who is competent to act in that capacity and whom I have accordingly engaged with the Bishop's consent, for that purpose. The expense of this appointment will be temporary only, as I hope soon to be able to dispense with the necessity of it by acquiring a sufficient knowledge of the oriental language to enable me to communicate with the natives. The various tongues which are spoken here cause no small impediment to the Missionary in the commencement of his labors. This is especially the case with Jerusalem, which seems to be the seat of every religion as well as every language.

The Hebrew and Greek are here living tongues, in addition to which there are the Arabic, Turkish, Coptic, Armenian, German, Spanish and Italian languages. The two latter are at present my principal medium of communication. To the above list may be added the English, which in connection with the Anglican church and our own mission, will hence-forth, with God's blessing be permanently established in the Holy City. Our dispensary may now be considered to be in full operation, as far as the means at our disposal and the nature of the circumstances permit. Since my last report, i.e. during March, April and May, I calculated that I have seen one thousand patients, more than a half of which number are regularly entered as dispensary-patients. I attend daily at the consultation room from 8 to 11 in the morning, with Mr. Bergheim, excepting Sundays. The number of patients seen every day varies from 10 to 30. They are admitted separately into the consultation room, where their names and symptoms and remedies prescribed are entered into a Register. At the expiration of the time I go out to visit patients at their own houses who are unable to attend in person, leaving Mr. Bergheim to dispense the prescriptions order for the day. These together with the other prescriptions from the out-door patients frequently keep him hard at work into a late hour in the evening.

It would be satisfactory to me to have it in my power to present to the committee in a tabular form the number of patients that have been admitted into the Dispensary with the details of their diseases and the cases which have been cured or received relief from the treatment adopted. But not only is the period in question too limited for such a statement; there are other circumstances arising from the peculiar character and habits of the patients themselves which would always render similar calculations both difficult and uncertain. The natives of this country of all classes, have no notion whatever of medical treatment. They take medicine as a kind of charm, which loses all its virtue unless immediately successful. With this impression they can scarcely ever be made to follow an exact and regular course of treatment, such especially as is required in chronic diseases of which the great majority of medical practice consists. If their extravagant expectations are not at once realized, they quickly lose all confidence in the reedy and either set out in quest of some other nostrum, or if they again make their appearance at the dispensary, attend in a very irregular manner. Their faith in strange and absurd remedies is unbounded. The boldest of our English quacks would stare with amazement at hearing of Elephant's fat, woman milk, the urine of a male cat and the horn of the Cerastes Snake, seriously recommended as infallible remedies in pulsses, pleurisies [sic.], obstructions, fevers and a number of other disorders. The reverence approaching to adoration, which was paid to Physicians in the past, is founded upon the supposition that he is the possessor of such secret charms and magical powers. These are not the materials from which medical returns can be drawn up. A hospital only can furnish data for satisfactory conclusions of that nature. For the present I must confine myself to general observations of the diseases most prevalent in the country.

Here as everywhere the diseases which most commonly prevail are chronic, and as might be expected this more especially the case in a poor, ill-fed, ill-clothed and badly lodged population. Of the acute forms of diseases intermittent fevers are most frequent arising principally from the bad water, which consists entirely of rain water collected during the rainy season and preserved in wells and tanks. As little or no attention is paid to the cleanliness of these reservoirs the water acquires deleterious properties and becomes the chief cause of ague. This complaint attacks all classes and all ages. It is not uncommon to see infants at the breast as well as their mothers suffering under regular attacks of intermittent fever. Foul air produced by want of sewers and the filthy state of the streets and houses, is, as stated in my last report, another futile cause of the same diseases. The prevalence of this complaint in so ill-conditioned a population lays the foundation of those visceral obstructions and enlargements and dropsical affections which are the most common chronic diseases of the country. At least two thirds of the patients which have come under my observation in this manner children of a tender age are often met with suffering from the same causes, with pale faces and swollen bellies, reminding me of the sickly population of the Pontini marshes. As these unfortunate beings live under the constant influence of the same predisposing and exciting causes, it is extremely difficult to afford them permanent relief by medical treatment.

The other forms of fever which I have most often met with are Typhus and Bilious fever. When these make their appearance in a family they generally attack every member of it, and give rise to scenes of appalling misery and suffering. It is under such circumstances that the care and attention of a physician are followed by the most signal and gratifying results. By the administration of proper remedies and suitable nourishment, by enforcing cleanliness and ventilation and by a diligent watchfulness of the patients I have been enabled to rescue many individuals and in some instances whole families from certain death. One case which occurred to me I have taken the liberty of relating. It took place in a Jewish family consisting of a young married couple a young infant at the breast and their aged parents. The husband was attacked with typhus fever of an aggravated character and under the most unfavorable circumstances. The family was living in a state of squalid poverty in a small and damp dwelling surrounded with filth vermin and a viscous atmosphere. After a dangerous illness of fifteen days the disease took a favourable turn and the patient was becoming convalescent when an imprudence in diet occasioned a relapse and brought on a renewal of the symptoms. By great care and watchfulness these were subdued and the patient was again restored to convalescence. At this period his wife was attacked with the same disease, and shortly afterwards her infant. The only attendant which now remained to act as nurse and attend upon the family was the aged mother, who herself then caught the complaint and was obliged to take to her bed at a time when her service had become most necessary. During her illness her old husband also caught the fever and was laid up in a separate building, and thus was the whole family laboring under the same fearful disease and destitute of all attendance and the necessaries of life. It became necessary for Mr. Bergheim and myself to act as nurses and to administer the medicines with our own hands, until after repeated applications to the Synagogue we at last obtained some attendance, but which was very insufficient. One day we had entered their miserable dwelling, but found the old mother missing from her bed, which consisted of a dirty mattress on the floor. At first I thought that she had died in the night and been removed – but on looking round the room I discovered the patient lying in a deep and dark recess in the wall, covered with a straw-mat, in a state of stupor. There was a strong stench of burning in the room which I found to issue from a pan of charcoal near the recess which had set fire to the straw mat which served as a covering to the bed. The fire had already reached the bedding which was signed by it, and would quickly have set it in flames had we not providentially entered in time to extinguish it. Nothing could have saved the poor creature from a dreadful death as there was no attendant in the house and the other invalids were in another room and incapable of rendering assistance had they known it to be required. The whole of this family recovered and by God's blessing were restored to health. It was but the other day that I met the young mother with her infant both looking better and cleaner than usual.

Diseases of the eye are very common in this climate, especially chronic ophthalmia, ulcers and opacity of the cornea. I am persuaded that poor and scanty diet is the chief cause of these afflictions, aggravated by want of cleanliness. Much benefit is to be claimed from medical treatment in these cases, but owing to the want of perseverance and skillfulness in the patients in the application of the remedies, it is much short of what it ought to be. Cataract is also very common, but as the operation for cataract requires both a previous and subsequent treatment it would be unsafe to attempt it until a proper ward for the reception of those cases shall have been provided.

Since the beginning of this month, bilious diarrhea and dysentery have been very prevalent. They are to be attributed to the extreme heat we have experienced and to the immoderate use of fruit such as orange and the young almonds and apricots and raw vegetables. Some of our mission have suffered but only very slightly from these complaints. Among other patients I may mention a Jew named Lazar, a sacrificer[sic.] of the German synagogue who is now recovering from a long and dangerous attack of dysentery. I mention his case more particularly as I understand that he is an Inquirer and favourably disposed to Xtianity[sic.]. His gratitude and that of his wife, who was also attacked with the same complaint, knows no bounds.

Also my patients lie principally among the Jewish population, my practice is not altogether confined to them. During the unusual concourse of pilgrims which were assembled this Easter at Jerusalem, from every country under heaven I had many patients of all classes and of all communities. I have particularly been called in to visit at the Greek convents both of monks and Nuns, and have been permitted in many instances to be the instrument of relief. Among the Greek Priests I have been fortunate enough to meet with some of superior attainments and amiable character, who are disposed to cultivate a friendly intercourse with us. But I am particularly pleased with what I have seen of the Armenians. They are interesting as individuals and as a religious society they seem to be less tainted with gross error and superstition than the other eastern churches…

and the medicines prescribed by the medical officer administered, at the hours prescribed, and that no food or medicine except such as ordered by the medical officers allowed to be taken by the patients. In summer the wards must be ready for the visit of the medical officer at 7 a.m. and in winter at 7.30 a.m.

2. Each head nurse will be responsible to the superintendent for the linen entrusted to her care entering in a book kept for the purpose, the articles of clothing etc. received by her from the Matron and those given back when soiled to be washed.
3. She will receive from the kitchen the food brought up to her ward by the porter or cook, and the medicines brought from the Dispensary and will alone be responsible for their due administration.
4. She will see that the patients when admitted are washed or bathed (subject to instruction from the medical officers) and that they are at once dressed in the Hospital clothing, their own clothes being taken from them and kept in a safe place until their owners are discharged, when they will be returned.
5. The head nurses will request the patients who come under their care to hand over any money or valuables they may possess for safe keeping and will warn them that unless such things are placed in the custody of the steward, the Hospital will not be in any degree accusable for them if lost.
6. The head nurses will see that the under nurses of their respective wards perform their duties satisfactorily and the under nurses will understand that they are to act under the orders of the head nurses who are responsible to the superintendent for them.
7. The head nurses will attend the morning prayers of the Hospital, will accompany the medical officers round their respective wards and receive from them instructions as to the dressings, taking of temperatures, medicines, diet etc. They will each [be] allowed two hours absence for recreation every day, and on Sundays [the] opportunity of attending the divine Service, but they must never all be absent from the Hospital at the same time, except for attendance at Sunday morning Service.

London Society for Promoting Christianity Amongst the Jews
Mission Hospital
Nurses Routine

Night Duty

	Summer	Winter
On duty	7. p.m.	9.0 p.m.
Off duty and supper	7. a.m.	7.30 a.m.
Bed	8. a.m.	go out 8 a.m.
Rise	3.30 p.m.	Bed 11.30 a.m.
Breakfast	4. p.m.	Rise 7.30 p.m.
Off duty for 2½ hours	4.30 p.m.	Breakf. 8. p.m.

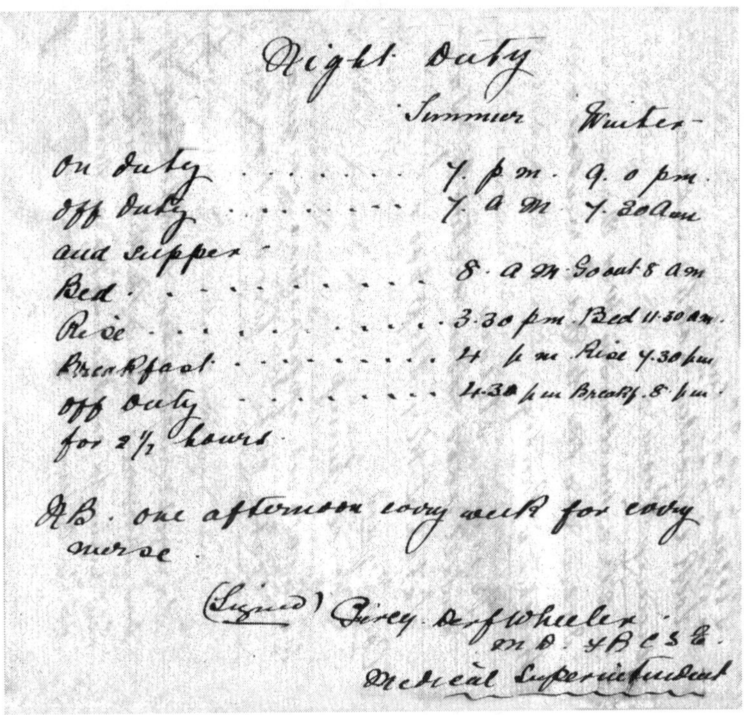
Night Duty

	Summer	Winter
On duty	7. p m.	9. 0 pm.
Off duty	7. a m	7. 30am
and supper		
Bed	8. a m.	Go out 8 am
Rise	3.30 pm.	Bed 11.30 am.
Breakfast	4 p m	Rise 7.30 pm
Off duty	4.30 p m	Breakf. 8. pm.
for 2½ hours		

N.B. one afternoon every week for every nurse.

(Signed) Percy d'Erf Wheeler
M.D. FRCSE.
Medical Superintendent

Figure 19 - Nurses "Night duty"

Day Duty

	Summer	Winter
Rise	5. a.m.	5.30 a.m.
Breakfast	6.30 a.m.	6. a.m.
On duty 1 to take over night duty cases & get ward ready.		
1½ hour	6. a.m.	6.30 a.m.
Ready for doctor	7.30 a.m.	8. a.m.
Patients dinner	11.30 a.m.	11.30 a.m.
Nurses do.	12 a.m.	12 a.m.
On duty	2. p.m.	1. p.m.
Off duty for 1 hour	5. p.m.	3. p.m.
On duty	6. p.m.	5. p.m.
Supper	8. p.m.	8. p.m.
Bed	9.30 p.m.	9.30 p.m.

NB. One afternoon [off] every week for every nurse.

(Signed) Percy d'Erf Wheeler
Medical Superintendent

NOTES

Introduction

1. Carmel, Alex, 'Activities of the European Powers in Palestine 1799-1914', *Asian and African Studies*, 19 (1985), pp. 43-92.
2. More about the Restoration of the Jews see: Vereté, Meir, 'The Restoration of the Jews in the Protestant Thought in England during the Years 1790-1840', *Zion*, 33 (1968), pp. 145-179 [Hebrew]; Kark, Ruth, 'Millenarism and Agricultural Settlement in the Holy Land in the Nineteenth Century', *Journal of Historical Geography*, 9 (1983), pp. 46-62.
3. On him see: Perry, Yaron, *British Mission to the Jews in Nineteenth-Century Palestine* (London, 2003), pp. 12-15.
4. Nicolayson (Hans Nicolajsen) was born on June 1, 1803. In 1821 he moved to Berlin and joined a seminary for missionaries. Two years later he was sent to London and spent two years in the Society's training centre in Stansted. After completing his studies in 1825 he was sent to Jerusalem, spent there several years, left due to the political turbulence in the area and return permanently after the Egyptian conquer. Nicolayson headed the London Jews Society in Palestine till his death in 1856. More about him see: Perry: *British Mission*, pp. 21-27; Nicolayson, John, 'Mittheilungen für eine Skizze der Geschichte der englischen Mission und des evangelischen Bisthums zu Jerusalem', *Zions-Bote*, 1 (1852), pp. 6-16; Nicolayson's Journal 1833-1856, in: Archive of the Israeli Trust of the Anglican Church (London Jews Society), Jerusalem (ITAC).
5. Nicolayson: 'Mittheilungen', p. 8.
6. Cumming, James Elder, 'Notes on Medical Mission', *The Church of Scotland Home and Foreign Missionary Record,* 1 October 1879, pp. 492-494. Rev. Dr Cumming, a Scottish Minister and scholar who wrote several works concerning the theory of mission.

35. Amar and Lev: *Physicians,* pp. 74-93; Amar, Zohar, *The history of medicine in Jerusalem* (Oxford, 2002), pp. 69-80.
36. Levy: *The History*, pp. 133-135. For further details on the Municipal Hospital see: Greenberg, Zalman, 'The Turkish Municipal Hospital in Jerusalem', *Cathedra*, 78 (1995), pp. 49-64 [Hebrew].
37. On the medicinal substances which were used by the inhabitants of Jerusalem until the beginning of the nineteenth century, see: Lev, Efraim, 'Medical Materials in Jerusalem from the 10th to the 18th Centuries', in: Z. Amar, E. Lev and J. Schwartz (eds.), *Medicine in Jerusalem Throughout the Ages* (Tel Aviv, 1999), pp. 51-78 [Hebrew].
38. Regarding quinine, see: Amar and Lev: *Physician*, p. 189.
39. See e.g., Lewis, A. William, *A Complete Dictionary of the Whole Materia Medica* (London, 1810).
40. In this connection, see: Tobler: *Beitrage*, pp. 16; Amar, Zohar and Lev, Efraim, 'Traditional Medicinal Substances in Jerusalem According to Titus Tobler', *Harefuah* 138 (2000), pp. 604-607 [Hebrew]; Lev, Efraim, *Medicinal Substances in Jerusalem from Early Times to Present Day* (Oxford, 2003), pp. 109-113.
41. Several sources from the 18th century refer to 'the Hospital of St. Helena' which was a hostel for the poor and a 'thekia' (a sort of soup-kitchen). See: Horn, Elzar, 'Ichnographiae Monumentorum Terrae Sanctae', in: E. Hoade and B. Bagatti (eds.), *Studium Biblicum Franciscanum*, No.15. (Jerusalem, 1962), pp. 191-193; Hasselquist, Friedrich, *Voyages and Travels in the Levant* (London, 1866), p. 135.
42. Freidin, Israel, 'Bikur Holim Perushim in Jerusalem – From Society to Hospital', *Cathedra*, 23 (1983), pp. 117-140 [Hebrew].
43. Benayahu, Meir, *Essays on Medicine by Rabbi Rephael Mordecai Malki* (Jerusalem, 1988), pp. 58-68 [Hebrew].
44. Tobler: *Beitrage*, pp. 12-15; Tobler, Titus, *Denkblätter aus Jerusalem* (Konstanz, 1853), pp. 403-404.
45. See in introduction to Horn: 'Ichnographiae', pp. 6-7.
46. Levy: *The History*, pp. 12-18.
47. Horn: 'Ichnographiae', pp. 176-178.
48. See, e.g.: Arce: 'Miscelanea', I, pp. 117-120, 324-325; Schur, Nathan, 'Franciscan Physicians and Pharmacists in Jerusalem', in: Z. Amar, E. Lev and J. Schwartz (eds.), *Medicine in Jerusalem throughout the Ages* (Tel Aviv, 1999), pp. 99-101.
49. Bagatti, Battista, 'Father Anthony Manzazi of Cuna (1650–1729), Inventor of the Balm of Jerusalem', *Franciscan Studies*, 6 (1946), pp. 250–361; Cirelli, A., *Gli Annali di Terra Sante* (Karachi, 1918), p. 219.
50. Horn: 'Ichnographiae', pp. 176-181.
51. Hasselquist: *Voyages*, p. 135.

52. Seetzen, J. Ulrich, *Reisen durch Syrien Palästina, etc.* (Berlin, 1854), II, pp. 205-206.
53. Arce: 'Miscelanea', III, pp. 418-427.
54. Schur: 'Franciscan', p. 104.
55. Amar, Zohar and Lev, Efraim, 'An Early Glimpse at Western Medicine in Jerusalem 1700-1840: The Case of the Jews and the Franciscans, Medical Activity', *Vesalius*, 11(2) (2005), pp. 81-87.
56. Schur: 'Franciscan', p. 104. The Franciscan medical institution appear in this chapter since they were not consider as a modern medical institute in the second half of the nineteenth century and therefore are not relevant to the chapter on the hospitals.
57. Amar and Lev: *Physicians*, pp. 71-74. See also the list of physicians in Jerusalem, ibid., pp. 103-116.
58. Heim: *Tobler*.
59. Tobler: *Beitrage*.
60. Ibid., pp. 14-15. In 1853 Tobler published his book: *Denkblätter aus Jerusalem* [Recollections of Jerusalem], which was based on his final visit to the city. One chapter of the book gives a detailed description of the local medical institutions in Jerusalem, together with an account of the establishment of certain modern medical institutes.
61. Levy: *The History*; Kass: 'Western'.
62. Tobler: *Beitrage*, pp. 12, 17.
63. Ibid., p. 16. See the complete list and its analysis in: Amar and Lev: '*The Traditional*', and in: Lev: *Medicinal Substances*, pp. 109-112.
64. The translations of the following paragraphs from Tobler's book have been dealt with in: Stern, Shimon, 'A Description of Medical Conditions in mid-19th-Century Jerusalem', in: Z. Amar, E. Lev and J. Schwartz (eds.), *Medicine in Jerusalem throughout the Ages* (Tel Aviv, 1999), pp. 107-127 [Hebrew]; Lev, Efraim and Amar, Zohar, 'The End of the Traditional Medicine in Jerusalem According to the Swiss Physician Titus Tobler (1806-1877)', *Canadian Bulletin for the History of Medicine*, 21 (2004), pp. 159-180.
65. Cunningham, Andrew and Williams, Perry (eds.), *The Laboratory Revolution in Medicine* (Cambridge, 1992). pp. 1-13.
66. Tobler: *Beitrage*, pp. 57-58.
67. Ibid., pp. 38-39.
68. Ibid., p. 32; Masterman asserts that 'Cholera appears in severe epidemics at intervals, with an enormous mortality'. He adds a significant sentence: 'In nothing does the fatalism of the ignorant natives appear more prominently than in their attitude towards this disease. In spite of all warning, they will wash the clothes of cholera patients in the village water-supply'. He then describes the Tiberias

epidemic of 1902: 'many of the people could not be induced to drink the boiled water freely and liberally supplied to them by the resident Scottish doctors, but used this for washing their clothes and drank of the sewage-infected lake-water at their doors'; Masterman: *Hygiene*, pp. 15-16; see also: Masterman, Ernest William Gurney, 'The cholera epidemic of last autumn in Palestine', *St. Bartholomew's Hospital Journal*, 10 (1903), pp. 62-63, 91-92.

69. Tobler: *Beitrage*, p. 45.
70. Ibid., p. 44; Masterman regarded 'Infantile diarrhoea and dysentery' as the cause of many deaths, see: Masterman: *Hygiene*, p. 23.
71. Tobler: *Beitrage*, p. 45.
72. Ibid., p. 39; Masterman added years later that 'Erysipelas is by no means uncommon among the town-dwellers, many cases contracting infection at site of the "issues" the people make and keep permanently open on their arms and elsewhere with the idea of benefiting their chronic eye-diseases', see: Masterman: *Hygiene*, p. 16.
73. Tobler: *Beitrage*, p. 24.
74. Ibid., p. 47, Masterman mentions that Hysteria was common among 'members of the Jewish race' see: Masterman: *Hygiene*, p. 18.
75. Tobler: *Beitrage*, p. 35.
76. Ibid., p. 37; Masterman reports that 'Eye diseases are, and probably always have been, very prevalent in the Holy Land'. He then goes on to detail the different diseases and symptoms, see: Masterman: *Hygiene*, pp. 20-22.
77. Tobler: *Beitrage*, p. 40.
78. Ibid., pp. 32-35; Malaria and its causes were extensively described by Masterman seventy years later from a more experienced and knowledgeable position (i.e., after germ theory and the laboratory revolution). See: Masterman: *Hygiene*, pp. 13-15. Malaria continued to be a common disease in Jerusalem well into the 20th century. See: Cropper, John, 'The Malaria fevers of Jerusalem and their prevention', *Journal of Hygiene*, 5 (1905), pp. 460-466. Masterman, Ernest William Gurney, 'Notes on some tropical diseases of Palestine', *Journal of Hygiene*, 13 (1913), pp. 49-62; 14 (1914), pp. 1-11. Muehlens, Peter, 'Bericht über eine Malaria Expedition nach Jerusalem', *Zentralbl. f. Bakt.*, 69 (1913), pp. 41-85. Yekutiel, Perez, 'Masterman, Muehlens and Malaria, Jerusalem 1912-1913', *Korot*, 12 (1996-1997), pp. 107-123.
79. Tobler: *Beitrage*, pp. 47-54; for his part, Dr Masterman writes: 'Leprosy is not a common disease but it infects all classes – Moslems, Jews and Christians: there are in all Palestine not more, perhaps, than

250 lepers, most of them segregated in Jerusalem'. He gives additional useful information in: Masterman: *Hygiene*, pp. 17-18.

80. Tobler: *Beitrage*, pp.25-32. Seventy years later Masterman reports: 'Plague has not occurred in epidemic form in Palestine since the first third of the nineteenth century, though sporadic cases have been detected and isolated at the ports; in earlier ages it swept the land with terrible effect', see: Masterman: *Hygiene*, p. 16.
81. Tobler: *Beitrage*, p. 36.
82. Ibid., p. 39; 'Acute rheumatism is fairly common', asserted Masterman seventy years later, 'and is responsible for a large proportion of the cases of valvular diseases of the heart', see: Masterman: *Hygiene*, p. 16.
83. Tobler: *Beitrage*, p. 25.
84. Ibid., p. 41. Decades later Masterman writes, 'Tetanus occurs occasionally... The Turkish Government, through the local authorities, assists all such cases, when needing financial help, to go Egypt or to Constantinople for treatment...', see: Masterman: *Hygiene*, p. 16.
85. Tobler: *Beitrage*, pp. 35-36.
86. Ibid., p. 58.
87. Ibid., p. 41.
88. Ben Maimon, Moses, *On Asthma*, S. Muntner (ed.) (Jerusalem, 1965) [Hebrew]; Dr Masterman later states, 'With regard to non-tubercular lung diseases, spasmodic asthma is very prevalent in Jerusalem', see: Masterman: *Hygiene*, p.19.
89. Tobler: *Beitrage*, p. 45.
90. Ibid., p. 41.
91. Ibid., p. 31.
92. Ibid., pp. 41-42.
93. Ibid., p. 36.
94. Ibid., p. 41. Masterman similarly avers that 'Various forms of Idiocy and Insanity are by no means uncommon, but suicide is distinctly rare', see: Masterman: *Hygiene*, pp. 42.
95. Tobler: *Beitrage*, p. 25.

English Mission Hospitals

1. See: Perry: *British Mission*, pp. 19-20.
2. *Jewish Expositor and the Friends of Israel*, X (1825), pp. 13-17, Lewis to London, 28.5.1824.
3. More about him see: Perry: *British Mission*, pp. 20-23, 27-28.

4. *Missionary Herald, American Board of Foreign Missions*, 23 (February 1827), pp. 34-35.
5. The Governor of Damascus, who had entered his position in 1822, imposed heavy taxes that aroused the anger of the inhabitants of the country. The revolt conducted against him, centred in Shechem and Jerusalem, went on until 1826. In 1825, he went out to the region himself, and the missionaries in Jerusalem were caught up in the midst of this event. The revolt was suppressed with the help of the Governor of Acre. On this, see mainly: Spyridon, S.N., 'Annals of Palestine 1821-1841', *Journal of the Palestine Oriental Society*, 18 (1938), pp. 63-152, in: *Extracts from Annals of Palestine 1821-1841, Manuscript – Monk Neophitos of Cyprus* (Jerusalem 1979), pp. 18-28.
6. *Missionary Herald*, 23 (February 1827), pp. 35-36.
7. *Jewish Expositor*, 11 (1826), pp. 183-186, Dalton: Diaries from Palestine 29.10.1825, Dalton from Tyre, 9.5.1825-18.5.1825; Ibid. 12 (1827), p. 26.
8. See: Perry: *British Mission*, p. 22.
9. *Jewish Expositor*, 12 (1827), pp. 143.
10. About 20 years later, the cemetery of the Protestant community was established nearby. A few years ago, Dalton's tombstone was transferred from the Greek cemetery to the nearby Protestant cemetery, where it lies today.
11. *Jewish Expositor*, 11 (1826), pp. 309-310.
12. Palestine Mission Journals by John Nicolayson III, 7.11. 1838, 3.12.1838, in the archive of the London Society for Promoting Christianity Amongst the Jews in Christ Church, Jerusalem (Christ Church)
13. ITAC, Correspondence from London, I: Cartwright from London, 2.8.1838.
14. Hyamson, Albert Montefiore, *The British Consulate in Jerusalem in Relation to the Jews of Palestine 1838-1914* (London, 1939), vol, 1, p. 9, Gerstmann to Young 15.5.1839 (FO-368/78).
15. McCaul was born and educated in Dublin and served as a missionary in Poland and Germany. In 1830 he settled in England and besides his position as a Professor of Theology at Kings College, he headed the educational institutions of the Society. From 1854 until his death, he was the Vice-President of the Society. See his obituary in: *Jewish Intelligence - Monthly Account of the Proceedings of the London Society for Promoting Christianity Amongst the Jews* (January 1864), pp. 2-10.
16. Christ-Church: Nicolayson's Journals, III, 11.2.1830.

17. *Report of the London Society for Promoting Christianity Amongst the Jews*, 31 (1830), p. 72. This plan was first recorded by Nicolayson in his diary. See: Christ-Church: Nicolayson's Journal, III, 28.12.1838, 11.2.1839.
18. Olin, Stephan, *Travels in Egypt, Arabia Petraea, and the Holy Land* (New York, 1843), Vol 1, p. 106.
19. ITAC, Correspondence from London, I: Cartwright from London, 25.7.1839.
20. ITAC, London Committee Resolutions, Nos. M1329, M1330, M1337 (26.3.1841).
21. Bodleian Library, Oxford, Department of Western Manuscripts, Dep. Cmj, c.125: Lease agreements and the purchase of parts of the pharmacy building.
22. Ibid., Listings of leases from November 1843 till September 1857; ITAC, Jerusalem Local Committee Minutes Book, I, No. 57 (27.9.1842).
23. *Jewish Intelligence* (January 1847), p. 21: Macgowan from Jerusalem.
24. Archive of the British Foreign Office at the Public Record Office, London (FO), FO-78/625: Young in Jerusalem to Aberdeen in London, 31.1.1845; ibid.: The Chief Rabbis to Macgowan, 21.1.1845; ibid.: Macgowan to Young, 21.1.1845; ibid.: Macgowan to Young 22.1.1845.
25. ITAC, Collection of unclassified documents: Original letter of excommunication in Rashi script with a handwritten English translation alongside.
26. ITAC, Medical Reports 1842-1899, a handwritten journal of the Jerusalem hospital's directors.
27. *Fifty-two Years Medical Work in Jerusalem*, (London, 1896), pp. 39-42, in: St. Albans.
28. *Jewish Missionary Intelligence, the Monthly Record of the London Society for Promoting Christianity Amongst the Jews* (July 1897), p. 105: Detailed description of the building sections and their functions as addendum to the panoramic photograph of the hospital. See: ibid. (January 1898), pp. 8-9.
29. Bodleian, Dep. Cmj, d.25: Invitation to the inaugural events of the new hospital, signed by the head of the Jerusalem Mission, Hastings Kelk, and Percy d'Erf Wheeler, director of the hospital; ibid.: Programme of the inauguration ceremony.
30. On the stormy demonstrations and bans issued against the hospital see: FO-195/1984: A series of exchanges between John Dickson, British Consul in Jerusalem, and Philip Henry Wodehouse Currie, the Ambassador in Constantinople. On the guards stationed by the Jewish community leaders at the gates of the hospital to prevent

Jewish patients from entering the institution, see: FO-195/2028: d'Erf Wheeler to Dickson.

31. *Jewish Missionary Intelligence* (August 1897), p. 115: The decree was translated into English and signed by the Chief Rabbi.
32. Ibid (October 1893), p. 146. The population figures given in square brackets are taken from Ben-Arieh, Yehoshua, 'The Landscape of Palestine on the Eve of the Zionist Colonization,' in: I. Kolatt (ed.) *The History of the Jewish Community in Eretz-Israel since 1882: The Ottoman Period* (Jerusalem, 1989), pp. 75-141 [Hebrew].
33. *Jewish Missionary Intelligence* (May 1903), p. 71.
34. Bodleian, Dep. Cmj, d.64: Anderson to the Secretary of the London Jews Society, 2.7.1903.
35. *Jewish Missionary Intelligence* (June 1905), p. 84.
36. Ibid (June 1907), p. 93: Anderson's speech before the London Committee, 3.5.1907.
37. Ibid (May 1907), p. 68.
38. Bodleian, Dep. Cmj, d.60. The complete list is to be found in: Lev, Efraim and Perry, Yaron, 'The 1857 Inventory of Materia Medica of the British Hospital in Jerusalem', *Pharmaceutical Historian*, 32 (2002), pp. 40-45. The decipherment of the handwriting was done with the assistance of nineteenth century medical and pharmacological studies such as the *British Pharmacopoeia* 1858, 4th ed. (London, 1880); and Woodville, Wilson, *Medical Botany*, vols. I-II (London, 1819).
39. Ulman, Yesim Isil, 'The First Surgical Use of Chloroform in the Ottoman Empire', *The New History of Medicine Studies* 5 (1999), pp. 87-94.
40. Lewis: *A Complete*.
41. *British Pharmacopoeia*.
42. Duncan, Andrew, *The Edinburgh New Dispensatory* (Edinburgh, 1804).
43. Horn: 'Ichnographiae', p. 189.
44. Lev, Efraim, 'Healing with Animals in the Levant from 10th to 18th century', *Journal of Etnobiology and Ethnomedicine* 2(11) (2006), pp. 1-11.
45. ITAC, Medical diaries, August 1845, p. 112.
46. Amar and Lev: 'The Traditional'.
47. Tobler: *Beitrage*, p. 16.
48. Ibid., p. 62.
49. Lev, Efraim, 'Reconstructed *materia medica* of the Medieval and Ottoman al-Sham', *Journal of Ethnopharmacology*, 80 (2002), pp. 167-179.
50. Tobler: *Beitrage*, p. 62.
51. Lev, Efraim, *Medicinal Substances of the Medieval Levant* (Tel-Aviv, 2002), pp. 139-140 [Hebrew].
52. Tobler: *Beitrage*, pp. 17, 45, 62.
53. Watson, Gilbert, *Theriac and Mithridatium* (London, 1966).

54. Amar, Zohar, 'The Export of Theriac from the Land of Israel and its Uses in the Middle Ages', *Korot*, 12 (1996-1997), pp. 16-29 [Hebrew].
55. Lev: *Medicinal*, pp. 281-282.
56. Lev, Efraim, 'The Doctrine of Signature in the Medieval and Ottoman Levant', *Vesalius*, 8 (2002), pp. 1-10.
57. Lev: 'Healing'.
58. Lev, Efraim, 'Medicinal Exploitation of Inorganic Substances in the Levant in the Medieval and Early Ottoman Periods', *Adler Museum Bulletin*, 28 (2002), pp. 11-16.

The British Physicians

1. *Jewish Intelligence* (June 1847), p. 224: a report dated June 1847.
2. Ibid. (March 1841), p. 88.
3. After Chaplin had served for two years as director of the hospital, the Prince of Wales donated the sum of £15 to the relief fund. See: *Jewish Intelligence* (April 1863), p. 90.
4. Cumming: 'Notes', pp. 492-494.
5. Ibid.
6. *Jewish Intelligence* (March 1841), p. 88.
7. ITAC: London Committee Resolutions, Nos. M1329, M1330, M1337 (26.3.1841)
8. *Jewish Intelligence* (June 1842), p. 214.
9. Macgowan's first report to the committee in London, dated February 26, 1842, in *Jewish Intelligence* (May 1842), pp. 163-165.
10. Bodleian, dep. Cmj, c.125: Lease agreements and the purchase of parts of the pharmacy building.
11. *Jewish Intelligence* (September 1842), pp. 320-321.
12. Macgowan to London on July 1, 1842, in: *Jewish Intelligence* (September 1842), p. 316.
13. *Jewish Intelligence* (September 1842), pp. 318-319.
14. A letter dated July 29, 1843, in: *Jewish Intelligence* (October 1843), pp. 349-350.
15. From a letter written by Rev. Ferdinand Christian Ewald dated November 2, 1843, in: *Jewish Intelligence* (January 1844), pp. 23; (March 1844), pp. 79.
16. Ibid. (March 1845), p. 90.
17. *Ibid.*
18. Macgowan's letter dated October 30, 1849, in: *Jewish Intelligence* (January 1850), p. 10.
19. *Jewish Intelligence* (November 1850), pp. 373-375.

20. Sandford in a letter to London on March 9, 1847 in: *Jewish Intelligence* (May 1847), pp. 157-158. Richard Sandford, LAC, MRCS, was appointed by the London Jews Society as house surgeon to the Jerusalem hospital. He arrived in October 1846 and served under Macgowan until 1856.
21. *Jewish Intelligence* (June 1847), p. 224, a report dated June 1847.
22. Ibid. (November 1846), p. 406-407.
23. Ibid. (January 1847), p. 21.
24. Ibid. (April 1846), pp. 115-116.
25. Grajewski, Pinchas Ben Zion, 'Letter from Montefiore to the Rabbis of the Jewish Community', *In Memory of the First Zionists*, P. B-Z. Grajewski (ed.) (Jerusalem, 1928), Chapter 11, n.p. [Hebrew]. Shimon Fränkel trained in medicine in Munich, and before his arrival in Palestine served as a ship's doctor in the Dutch Navy.
26. Macgowan's report of March/April 1843, in: *Jewish Intelligence* (July 1843), p. 260.
27. Macgowan's report of May 31, 1843, in: *Jewish Intelligence* (August 1843), p. 287.
28. *Jewish Intelligence* (April 1846), p. 118.
29. For example: *Jewish Intelligence* (October 1846), p. 371; (November 1846), p. 409; (March 1847), p. 105; (May 1847), p. 153-155; (August 1847), p. 291; (October 1847), p. 359.
30. Lev, Efraim and Perry, Yaron, 'Dr Thomas Chaplin, Scientist and Scholar in Nineteenth-Century Palestine', *Palestine Exploration Quarterly,* 136 (2004), pp. 151-162.
31. Henry Crawford, in: *Jewish Intelligence* (April 1860), p. 106-107.
32. *Jewish Intelligence* (April 1860), pp. 106-107.
33. See his eulogy in: *Jewish Missionary Intelligence* (November 1904), p. 162. One may learn about his character as a congenial, kind-hearted, and courteous person from his eulogy in the quarterly journal of the Palestine Exploration Fund: 'His kindness of heart, or that combination of firmness and gentleness in his character which enabled him to win the respect and esteem of Christians, Moslems and Jews…', in: *Palestine Exploration Quarterly*, 37 (1905), p. 14.
34. *The Medical Register,* London (1863), p. 69; (1885), p. 219.
35. Lecture dated March 21, 1888, in: *Jewish Intelligence* (May 1888), pp. 65-69.
36. *Jewish Intelligence* (December 1865), p. 313.
37. All five children were baptized in Christ Church, Jerusalem. See: Christ Church: Baptisms Register: Emily Ada Sophia was baptized on March 29, 1868 (see: p. 43, No. 339); Alfred William was baptized on February 14, 1869 (see: p. 44, No. 348); Elizabeth Charlotte Maud

was baptized on October 16, 1870 (see: p. 47, No. 371) and died April 4, 1872; Janet Mabel was baptized on March 1, 1873 (see: p. 51, No. 406).

38. *Palestine Exploration Quarterly*, 37 (1905), p. 14.
39. Bodleian, Dep. Cmj, d.25: Report of T. Chaplin 1897.
40. *Palestine Exploration Quarterly*, 37 (1905), p. 16.
41. Chaplin, Thomas, *On Some Diseases Mentioned in the Bible* (London, 1902).
42. Preuss, Julius, *Biblical and Talmudic Medicine* (New York, 1983).
43. Much later, in 1920, Masterman wrote a monograph on the same theme, see: Masterman: *Hygiene*. He describes the medical situation in Palestine, the widespread diseases there, as well as explanations and modern identifications of illnesses and medical incidents recorded in the Bible.
44. *Palestine Exploration Quarterly*, 37 (1905), p. 15.
45. Chaplin: 'The Fevers', pp. 236-238, 256-269, 289-291.
46. Greenberg: 'The Earliest'; Levy: *The History*, pp. 33-34. Four years later Chaplin published another article which described Leuce case. See: Chaplin, Thomas, 'On the Case of Leuce', *Lancet*, 6 (1868), p. 656. Seventeen years later he published an article describing malarial typhoid. See: Chaplin, Thomas, 'On malarial typhoid fever', *Lancet*, 22 (1885), pp. 518-520.
47. Chaplin: 'The Fevers'.
48. Hansen, A. Gerald, 'On the Etiology of Leprosy', *Chirurgical Review,* 55 (1875), pp. 459-489.
49. Browne, Stanley George, 'The History of Leprosy', in: R.C. Hastings (ed), *Leprosy* (Edinburgh, London and New York, 1985), pp 1-14; Bryceson, Anthony and Pfaltzgraff, E. Roy, *Leprosy* (Edinburgh, London and New York, 1979), pp. 1-2.
50. Chaplin: *Diseases*, pp. 8-14.
51. Ibid., p. 9.
52. *Palestine Exploration Quarterly*, 37 (1905), pp. 15.
53. Levy: *The History*, pp. 128-129.
54. More about the hospital and Chaplin's part in its establishing see on pages 121-125.
55. Buchan, A., 'Remarks on the Climate of Jerusalem, from Observations made by Dr Thomas Chaplin for three years and four months, beginning November 1, 1863, and ending February 28, 1867', *Palestine Exploration Quarterly*, 3 (1872), pp. 19-30.
56. Chaplin, Thomas, 'Observations on the Climate of Jerusalem', *Palestine Exploration Quarterly*, 15 (1883), pp. 8-40.

57. Goldreich, Yair, *The Climate of Israel: Observations, Research and Applications* (New York, 2003), p. 19.
58. *Palestine Exploration Quarterly,* 37 (1905), p. 15.
59. Ibid., p. 14. Obadiah di Bertinoro journeyed to Jerusalem in 1488 and during the four years he spent in the city, he acted as "Chief of all the Rabbis of Jerusalem." Among his significant works was the commentary on the Mishna. See: Hartum, Menachem Emanuele and David, Aabrham, *From Italy to Jerusalem: Letters of Rabbi Obadiah mi-Bartenura* (Jerusalem, 1997) [Hebrew].
60. Maimonides = Rabbi Moses ben Maimon (1135-1204) was born in Cordoba and later practiced as a physician in Egypt. He was considered one of the greatest scholars of his time, and wrote highly important Halachic and exegetical works.
61. Warren, Charles and Conder, Claude Reigneir, *The Survey of Western Palestine, Jerusalem* (London, 1884).
62. Ibid., pp. 261-262.
63. Arabic script with heavy, angular lettering characteristic of the seventh century CE, but no longer in use except for decorative purposes.
64. Chaplin, Thomas, 'Letter from Dr Chaplin', *Palestine Exploration Quarterly*, 5 (1873), pp. 155-156.
65. Kloner, Amos and Zissu, Boaz, *The Necropolis of Jerusalem in the Second Temple Period* (Jerusalem, 2003), pp. 121-122 [Hebrew].
66. Ibid.
67. Sayce, A. Henry, 'The Ancient Hebrew Inscription in the Pool of Siloam', *Palestine Exploration Quarterly*, 13 (1881), pp. 282-285.
68. Warren, Charles, 'Copy of Letter Lost at es-Salt', *Palestine Exploration Quarterly*, 1 (1869), pp. 13-14.
69. According to the archeologists Dr Magen Broshi, Dr Gabi Barkay and Dr Boaz Zissu (Personal communication).
70. Chaplin, Thomas, 'The Site of Ebenezer', *Palestine Exploration Quarterly*, 20 (1888), pp. 263-265.
71. *Encyclopedia Biblica* (Jerusalem, 1956), vol. I, pp. 49-50.
72. *Jewish Missionary Intelligence* (July 1898), p. 100.
73. 'An Address Given at the Annual Breakfast, 6.5.1898', in: *Jewish Missionary Intelligence* (July 1898), pp. 100-101.
74. *Palestine Exploration Quarterly*, 37 (1905), p. 14.
75. From a speech given at the annual conference of the London Jews Society on May 6, 1886, in: *Jewish Intelligence* (June 1886), p. 107.
76. Anon., 'Obituary Notice, Dr Percy d'Erf Wheeler, F.R.C.S.' *Palestine Exploration Quarterly*, 77 (1945), pp. 54-55; 'Royal College of Surgeons', *The Times* (Friday, May 16, 1884), p. 4.

77. For more of him see: Perry, Yaron and Lev, Efraim, 'Dr Percy Charles Edward d'Erf Wheeler (1859-1944). A Notable Medical Missionary of the Holy Land', *Journal of Medical Biography* (in press).
78. Perry, Yaron and Lev, Efraim, 'Nineteenth Century Medical Activities of the London Society for Promoting Christianity Amongst the Jews, in the Holy Land', *Medical History*, 47 (2003), pp. 67-88.
79. *Jewish Intelligence* (August 1889), p. 113.
80. *Jewish Missionary Intelligence* (January 1898), pp. 8-9, a detailed description of the building sections and their functions, as an addendum to the panoramic photograph of the hospital.
81. Bodleian, Dep. Cmj, d.25: Invitation to the inauguration events of the new hospital, signed by the head of the Jerusalem Mission, Hastings Kelk, and Percy d'Erf Wheeler, director of the hospital.
82. *Jewish Missionary Intelligence* (August 1893), p. 126; 'Marriages', *The Times* (Thursday July 20, 1893), p. 1.
83. 'Killed in Action', *The Times* (Friday, July 27, 1917), p. 1; Anon.: 'Wheeler's obituary'.
84. *Jewish Missionary Intelligence* (June 1906), p. 83.
85. St. Albans, Applications and Appointments, A, No. 171.
86. *Jewish Missionary Intelligence* (June 1906), p. 83.
87. Ibid. (January 1898), p. 15; (July 1891), p. 108.
88. Ibid. (June 1906), pp. 87-88; (June 1908), pp. 86-87.
89. Ibid. (June 1891), pp. 93-95.
90. Ibid. (June 1906), pp. 87-88.
91. Wheeler, Percy d'Erf, 'Jerusalem Notes: Hospital Cleanings', *Jewish Missionary Intelligence* (June 1907), pp. 86-87.
92. Wheeler, Percy d'Erf, 'Visitation of the Sick in Jerusalem', *Jewish Missionary Intelligence* (November 1901), pp. 168-170.
93. Perry: *British Mission*, p. 184.
94. *Jewish Missionary Intelligence* (September 1909), p. 137.
95. Perry, Yaron and Lev, Efraim, 'Ernest William Gurney Masterman, British Physician and Scholar in the Holy Land', *Palestine Exploration Quarterly*, 138, 2(2006), pp. 133-146.
96. *Jewish Missionary Intelligence* (March 1910), p. 34.
97. 'Testimonial to Dr Percy d'Erf Wheeler', *Jewish Missionary Intelligence* (May 1910), p. 77.
98. Ibid.
99. Ibid. (1919), pp. 143-146.
100. Ibid. (1921), p. 181.
101. *Palestine Exploration Quarterly*, 39 (1907), pp. 246-247; 40 (1908), pp. 4-5, 86-87; 41 (1909), pp. 159-160.
102. Lev and Perry: 'Chaplin'.

103. Perry and Lev: 'Masterman'.
104. Anon.: 'Wheeler's obituary'.
105. C.F.G. Masterman was one of the principal builders of the British national health insurance system and the first chairman of the insurance commission (whose function in days to come were taken over by the Ministry of Health). Ernest Masterman derived his third Christian name – Gurney – from his mother's family. See: *British Medical Journal* (April 17, 1943), p. 493.
106. *The UK Medical Directory* (1943), p. 2130.
107. On Johannes Zeller see: Reiche-Zeller, Lisl, *Johannes Zeller 1830-1902. Missionar in Palästina* (Stuttgart, 1987); Ben Arzi, Yossi, 'Johannes Zeller – a missionary to Nazareth and the Holy Land', *Cathedra*, 50 (1989), 73-97 [Hebrew]. On Gobat see: Thiersch, W.J. Heinrich, and Gobat, Samuel, *Samuel Gobat, Bishop of Jerusalem, His Life and Work* (London, 1884); Perry, Yaron, 'Gobat, Samuel (1799-1879), bishop in Jerusalem', *Oxford Dictionary of National Biography*, vol. 22, p. 537 (Oxford, 2004).
108. Three of the children were born and baptized in Jerusalem: Muriel Gladys (October 1900), Florence Isabel Joy (August 1902), and Sylvia Rosalind (1906). See: Christ Church: Baptisms Register.
109. *Jewish Missionary Intelligence* (March 1895), p. 34-35; (September 1896), p. 141. The Maxwell Fund was named after a young physician whose wish was to become a medical missionary among the Jews of the East. After his death (December 1894), his friends set up the Fund to support a medical missionary in his stead. Masterman was the 'Eustace Maxwell Memorial Missionary' for 12 years.
110. On the mission activities in Siloam village see: Perry: *British Mission*, p. 184.
111. On that mission society see mainly: Stock, Eugene, *The History of the Church Missionary Society: Its Environment, Its Men and Its Work*, 3 vols. (London, 1899).
112. *British Medical Journal* (April 17, 1943), p. 493; Anno., 'Obituary Notice, Masterman, Ernest William Gurney', *Palestine Exploration Quarterly*, 75 (1943), pp. 70-73.
113. One of these was head of the Palestine Exploration Fund in the Holy Land,
114. Anno.: 'Masterman's obituary'.
115. Ibid.
116. Ibid.
117. Hanauer, James Edward and Masterman, Ernest William Gurney, *Cook's Hand Book for Palestine and Syria* (London, 1907).

118. Masterman, Ernest William Gurney, 'Jerusalem outside the walls', *Jewish Missionary Intelligence* (November 1895), pp. 174-175, 192-195.
119. Ibid., p. 174.
120. Ibid. (April 1909), pp. 56-57: Masterman at a missionary meeting in London on February 12, 1909.
121. Ibid. (June 1914), pp. 86-88.
122. Ibid. (December 1899), p. 84.
123. Masterman, Ernest William Gurney, *The Deliverance of Jerusalem* (London, New York and Toronto, 1918).
124. Masterman, Ernest William Gurney, 'Palestine: its resources and suitability for colonization', *The Geographical Journal*, 50 (1917), pp. 12-26.
125. Masterman, Ernest William Gurney, 'The water supply of Jerusalem, ancient and modern', *The Biblical World*, 19 (1902), pp. 87-112.
126. Anno.: '*Masterman's obituary*'. More than forty years before Macalister wrote Masterman's obituary, he gave the *Palestine Exploration Quarterly* a different version of the events. According to his report, he himself visited the western shores of the Dead Sea on October 8, 1900, located the rock in question and gave orders to mark the water level. Macalister concludes this explicit description by saying that 'Dr. Masterman, of Jerusalem, accompanied me', see: *Palestine Exploration Quarterly*, 33 (1901), pp. 4-5. The mystery becomes compounded years later when, in another article: Underhill, H.W, 'Dead Sea levels and P.E.F. mark', *Palestine Exploration Quarterly*, 99 (1967), p. 45, the author states that the water level mark made in 1900 was done by 'Macalister, a doctor at the Mission hospital in Jerusalem'. Our assumption is that there was an inadvertent textual error in the article by Underhill, and that what apparently occurred was that Macalister and Masterman – 'the doctor at the Mission hospital in Jerusalem' visited the Dead Sea (just as they often went on tours around the country together) and marked the water level.
127. Masterman, Ernest William Gurney, 'Ein El-Feshkhah, El-Hajar El-Asbah, and Khurbat Kumran', *Palestine Exploration Quarterly*, 34 (1902), pp. 297-299; Masterman, Ernest William Gurney, 'Notes on some ruins and a rock-cut aqueduct in the wady Kumran', *Palestine Exploration Quarterly*, 35 (1903), pp. 264-267.
128. Masterman, Ernest William Gurney, *Studies in Galilee* (Chicago, 1909).
129. Masterman, Ernest William Gurney, 'The fisheries of Galilee', *Palestine Exploration Quarterly*, 40 (1908), pp. 40-51.
130. Macalister, Robert Alexander Stewart and Masterman, Ernest William Gurney, 'Occasional papers on the modern inhabitants of Palestine', *Palestine Exploration Quarterly*, 38 (1906), pp. 33-50, 110-114, 223-225, 286-291.

131. *Palestine Exploration Quarterly*, 37 (1905), pp. 48-61, 343-356.
132. Ibid., 38 (1906), pp. 33-50, 110-114, 223-225, 286-291.
133. Masterman, Ernest William Gurney, 'The trees and shrubs of the Holy Land', *Palestine Exploration Quarterly*, 39 (1907), pp. 66-67.
134. Masterman, Ernest William Gurney, 'Vine', *The International Standard Bible Encyclopedia* (ed. J. Orr) (Chicago, 1915).
135. Anno.: 'Masterman's obituary'.
136. Masterman, Ernest William Gurney, 'Miscellaneous notes made during a journey east and west of Jordan', *Palestine Exploration Quarterly*, 34 (1902), pp. 299-301.
137. Masterman, Ernest William Gurney, 'The recently-discovered aqueduct from the Virgins fountain', *Palestine Exploration Quarterly*, 34 (1902), pp. 35-38.
138. Masterman: '*Notes on some ruins*'.
139. Masterman, Ernest William Gurney, 'The site of Capernaum', *Palestine Exploration Quarterly*, 39 (1907), pp. 220-229.
140. Masterman, Ernest William Gurney, 'Chephirah of Benjamin', *Palestine Exploration Quarterly*, 39 (1907), pp. 64-65.
141. Macalister, Robert Alexander Stewart and Masterman, Ernest William Gurney, 'Diary of a visit to Safed', *Palestine Exploration Quarterly*, 39 (1907), pp. 91-130.
142. Masterman, Ernest William Gurney, 'The Galilee of Josephus, the positions of Gabara, Jotapata and Taricheae', *Palestine Exploration Quarterly*, 42 (1910), pp. 268-280.
143. Ein Gedy is a spring in the foothills of the Judean desert near the Dead Sea shore, where there are ruins of an early Bronze period temple, caves, and remains of a Jewish village and synagogue dating to the Second Temple and Byzantine periods. Masada is a fortress on a mountain-top in the Judean desert foothills near the Dead Sea shore. It was built by the Hasmonaeans, and was the last stronghold against the Romans during the Jewish revolt that ended in 73AD. Jebal Usdum is a large salt mountain on the south-western shore of the Dead Sea.
144. Masterman, Ernest William Gurney, 'Notes of a visit to Engedy, Masada, and Jebal Usdum', *Palestine Exploration Quarterly*, 40 (1908), pp. 229-244.
145. Masterman, Ernest William Gurney, 'A Greek inscription from a column at Damascus', *Palestine Exploration Quarterly*, 28 (1896), pp. 340-341.
146. Masterman, Ernest William Gurney, 'A Greek inscription from the Grand Mosque, Damascus', *Palestine Exploration Quarterly*, 28 (1896), pp. 224-225.

147. Masterman, Ernest William Gurney, 'Notes from Damascus', *Palestine Exploration Quarterly*, 29 (1897), pp. 147-148.
148. Masterman, Ernest William Gurney, 'The Damascus railways', *Palestine Exploration Quarterly*, 29 (1897), pp. 198-200.
149. Masterman, Ernest William Gurney, 'The water of Jacob's Well', *Palestine Exploration Quarterly*, 29 (1897), pp. 149-151.
150. Smith, a Scottish Bible scholar and Hebraist, was professor of Old Testament language, literature and theology in the United Free Church College of Glasgow and principal and vice-chancellor of the University of Aberdeen.
151. Smith, George Adam, *Historical Geography of the Holy Land* (London 1931).
152. Masterman, Ernest William Gurney, 'Two cases of spreading gangrene around the mouth occurring in adults', *St. Bartholomew's Hospital Report*, 27 (1891), pp. 205-210.
153. Masterman, Ernest William Gurney, 'Rodent ulcer', *St. Bartholomew's Hospital Report*, 29 (1893), pp. 189-201.
154. Masterman, Ernest William Gurney, 'A smallpox epidemic in Jerusalem', *St. Bartholomew's Hospital Journal* (November 1900), pp.19-21.
155. Masterman: 'The cholera'.
156. Masterman: 'Notes'.
157. Ibid.
158. Masterman, Ernest William Gurney, 'Hirudinea as human parasites in Palestine', *Parasitology*, 1 (1908), pp. 182-185.
159. Masterman, Ernest William Gurney, 'Haemoglobinuric fever in Syria, and some notes on the occurrence of the disease in Palestine', *British Medical Journal*, 1 (1906), pp. 314-315.
160. On Chaplin see: Lev and Perry: 'Chaplin'.
161. Chaplin: 'The Fevers', pp. 236-238, 256-269, 289-291.
162. Greenberg: 'The Earliest'; Levy: *The History*, pp. 33-34.
163. See for example: Chaplin: 'On malarial'.
164. Masterman, Ernest William Gurney, 'Notes and news', *Palestine Exploration Quarterly*, 37 (1905). A similar report was published a few years before as a thesis for M.D. degree at the University of Cambridge: Cropper: 'Malarial', pp. 47-57.
165. Bruenn, W. and Goldberg, L., 'Die Malaria Jerusalems und ihre Bekämpfung', *Zeitschrift für Hygiene und Infektionskrankheiten*, 75 (1913), pp. 209-235.
166. Wheeler, Percy d'Erf, 'Malaria', *Palestine Exploration Quarterly*, 39 (1907), pp. 246-247; 40 (1908) pp. 86-87; 41 (1909), pp. 159-160. A description of this disease was made by the Swiss physician Dr Titus Tobler. According to him, malaria was: 'One of the most common

diseases in the city. All the European physicians agreed that it appeared frequently all year round, but reached a peak in the spring. The disease struck everyone, including babies and nursing mothers. The fever appeared in its single, double, triple, and even quadruple form. The high temperature was not fatal'. See: Tobler: *Beitrage*, pp. 32-35. Tobler sought its cause in the 'consumption of uncooked fruits', and heard that it 'might be from poisonous vapor coming from the Dead Sea'. He indicated that a likely cause could well be the water kept in the dirty cisterns and pools. It should be mentioned that Tobler, as well as Dr Edward Macgowan, founder of the English Mission Hospital in Jerusalem, made their observations prior to the discovery of the malarial parasite by Alphonse Laveran (1849-1922) in 1880. The hypothesis that the vector for the parasite was the anopheles mosquito was advanced by Sir Patrick Manson (1844-1922) in 1894 and demonstrated by Sir Ronald Ross (1857-1932) in 1897. See: Harrison, Gordon, *Mosquitoes, Malaria and Man: A History of the Hostilities Since 1880* (New York, 1978), pp. 10, 33, 102-104. Macgowan asserted that dwelling near the Patriarch pool was unhealthy and susceptible to malaria. From a study he conducted Tobler concluded that 'there were a considerable number of cases of malaria near the pool, more than in other parts of the city'. He blames the vapour and not the quality of the drinking water. Tobler's observation of the epidemiological connection between the Patriarch's Pool and the incidence of cases of malaria in Jerusalem was remarkably perceptive for the time, being based on a statistical analysis of the distribution of the disease. High temperature was treated with large quantities of quinine (Tobler was critical of the quantities). The inhabitants used a 'traditional medication, which consisted of: apricot seeds, aniseed, rue, lemon juice and urine. They also used amulets, a vegetarian diet for 40 days and other magic'. See: Lev and Amar: 'The End'.

167. Masterman: 'Notes'.
168. Muelens: *Bericht.*
169. Cropper: 'Malarial'.
170. Masterman, Ernest William Gurney, 'The new public health service in Palestine', *Palestine Exploration Quarterly*, 54 (1922), pp. 148-153 (abstract of the 1921 Annual Report, Ministry of Health). A modern malaria expert, Perez Yekutiel, comments in an article on 'Masterman's emphasis on prevention' and his 'enthusiasm', which prompted him to continue the blood survey among patients of his hospital and dispensaries after Muehlens' departure in January 1913, in order to complete a full year. See: Yekutiel: 'Masterman'.

171. Masterman, Ernest William Gurney, 'Jerusalem from the sanitary point of view', *Home Words for Jerusalem* (1904).
172. Masterman, Ernest, William, Gurney, 'The history of the Jerusalem medicinal mission', *Home Words for Jerusalem*, 41 (February, 1911), in: *Jewish Missionary Intelligence* (January 1911), pp. 12-14; (December 1911), p. 186.
173. *Jewish Missionary Intelligence* (March 1910), p. 35; (May 1910), p. 74; (October 1910), p. 146; (December 1910), p. 178; (January 1911), pp. 12-14; (December 1911), p. 186; (January 1912), pp. 3-6; (July 1912), p. 100; (May 1913), pp. 71-73; (August 1913), p. 118; (November 1913), p. 175; (December 1913), p. 183; (February 1914), p. 25.
174. See for example: Chaplin: *Diseases.*
175. Masterman, Ernest William Gurney, 'Hygiene and disease in Palestine in modern and in biblical times', *Palestine Exploration Quarterly*, 50 (1918), pp. 13-20, 56-71, 112-119; 51 (1919), pp. 27-36.
176. Masterman: *Hygiene.* (Review in: *Tropical Disease Bulletin* (1920), 1585-1586, and in: *Lancet*, 2 (1919), p. 879.
177. Masterman: 'The new'.
178. Anno.: 'Masterman's obituary'.
179. Yekutiel: 'Masterman'.
180. Personal communication with various scholars of diverse institutions and fields.
181. Masterman, Ernest William Gurney, 'Observations on the Dead Sea levels', *Palestine Exploration Quarterly*, 34 (1902), pp. 155-167, 297-301, 406-407; 35 (1903), pp. 177-178; 36 (1904), pp. 83-95, 163-168, 280-281; 37 (1905), pp. 158-161; 39 (1907), pp. 302-304; 40 (1908), pp. 160-161; 41 (1909), pp. 68-70.
182. Masterman, Ernest William Gurney, 'Summary of observations on the rise and fall of the level of the Dead Sea. 1900-1913', *Palestine Exploration Quarterly*, 45 (1913), pp. 192-197.
183. See for example: Raz, Eli, *Dead Sea Book* (Jerusalem, 1993), pp. 61-62.
184. Masterman: *Hygiene.*
185. See for example: Lev and Amar: 'The End'.
186. Masterman: *Galilee*, p. VIII.
187. *Jewish Missionary Intelligence* (June 1899), p. 91.
188. Gidney, William Thomas, *History of the London Society for Promoting Christianity amongst the Jews* (London, 1908), p. 553.
189. *Repor:* 86 (March 1894) p. XI: Appointments, Removals of Missionaries from April 1, 1893 till March 31, 1894.
190. *Jewish Missionary Intelligence* (August 1900), p. 114.
191. Gidney: *History,* p. 554.

192. *Jewish Missionary Intelligence* (December 1899), p. 184, Anderson's speech at the London Jews Society's annual meeting.
193. Ibid. (June 1899), p. 91.
194. Ibid. (January 1916), p. 2.
195. Ibid. (1937), p. 70, Obituary.

Impact

1. On Bunsen see: Bunsen, Frances, *A Memoir of Baron Bunsen, Drawn Chiefly from Family Papers by his Widow Frances Bunsen*, 2 vols. (2nd ed.) (London, 1869); Ruppel, Hans-Rudolf (ed.), *Universeller Geist und gutter Europäer Christian Carl Josias von Bunsen 1791-1860* (Korbach, 1991). On the Bishopric in general, see: Schmidt-Clausen, Kurt, *Vorweggenommene Einheit. Die Gründung des Bistums Jerusalem in Jahre 1841* (Berlin-Hamburg, 1965); Abeken, Heinrich, *The Protestant Bishopric in Jerusalem: Its Origin and Progress. From the Official Documents Published by Command of His Majesty the King of Prussia and from other Authentic Sources* (London, 1847); Hechler, William Henry, *The Jerusalem Bishopric, 1841. Documents Chiefly Reprinted from a Copy of the Original German Account, 'Das Evangelische Bisthum in Jerusalem.' Geschichtliche Darlegung mit Urkunden* (Berlin, 1842; London, 1883); Lückhoff, Martin, *Anglikaner und Protestanten im Heiligen Land* (Wiesbaden, 1998); Perry, Yaron, 'Anglo-German Cooperation in the Nineteenth-Century Jerusalem: The London Jews Society and the Protestant Bishopric', *Jewish Culture and History*, 4 (2001), pp. 65-80.
2. Bodleian, Dep. Cmj, d.55, pp. 1-9; Hechler: *Bishopric*, appendix, p. 110, declaration of principle for the establishing of the Bishopric, 9.12.1841.
3. The son of a Jewish Rabbi, Alexander was born in Schönlanke in the Duchy of Posen. In 1820 he arrived in England, wandered from town to town, serving as teacher and Rabbi. In 1825 he had converted to Christianity, attached himself to the London Jews Society and worked for the Society as missionary all over Europe. More on Alexander, see: Perry, Yaron, 'Alexander, Michael Solomon (1799-1845), first bishop of the United Church of England and Ireland and of the Protestant Church of Germany in Jerusalem', *Oxford Dictionary of National Biography* (Oxford, 2004), vol. 1, pp. 681-683; Lambeth Palace Archive, London, MSS-3393-7, Alexander's Papers; St. Albans: A booklet in his memory, pp. 33-53, pp. 68-71; Corey, W. Muriel, *From Rabbi to Bishop, the Biography of the Right Reverend Michael Solomon Alexander, Bishop in Jerusalem* (London, [1956]), pp. 9-44.

4. Hechler: *Bishopric,* appendix, p.110, declaration of principle for the establishing of the Bishopric, 9.12.1841.
5. *Report,* 38 (1846), p. 46.
6. Thiersch: *Gobat,* p. 289.
7. Ibid., p. 216.
8. On Fliedner see: Carmel, Alex, 'Der Missionar Theodor Fliedner als Pionier deutscher Palästina-Arbeit', in G. Walter (ed.), *Jahrbuch des Instituts für Deutsche Geschichte* (Tel-Aviv, 1985), vol. XIV, pp. 191-220; Fliedner, Georg, *Theodor Fliedner. Sein Leben und Wirken,* 2 vols. (Kaiserswerth, 1908, 1910).
9. Sticker, D. Anna, *Theodor Fliedner and Nursing* (Düsseldorf, 1972).
10. Nightingale, Florence, *The Institution of Kaiserswerth on the Rhine* (London, 1851).
11. The new building for the 'Talitha Kumi' school outside the city walls was considered to be an educational breakthrough in Palestine. On the Deaconessen hospital see: *Bericht über die Diakonissen-Stationen im Morgenlande, Kaiserswerth, 1851-1899*, passim ; Schwake, Norbert, *Die Entwicklung des Krankenhauswesens der Stadt Jerusalem vom Ende des 18. bis zum Beginn des 20.Jahrhunderts* (Hezogenrath, 1983), vol. I, pp. 245-346; Levy: *The History*, pp. 103-110.
12. He was the son of Dr Carl Sandreczki of the British Church Missionary Society, who joined Fliedner and the 4 Deaconesses on their way in 1851 to Palestine. On Sandreczki see on pages 117-121.
13. Cohn, Erich, *Women in Jerusalem* (Unpublished manuscript: Chapter on the Deaconesses of Kaiserswerth, Second Draught, July 1994), based on *Bericht über die Diakonissen-Stationen im Morgenlande, Kaiserswerth 1851-1899.*
14. In 1905, for example, nine nurses worked in the hospital, which had treated that year 1108 in-patients. An average of 70 people visited the ward every day, each of whom stayed for three weeks or more.
15. Tobler: *Beitrage*, pp. 47-54.
16. Ibid.
17. Hansen: *Etiology*; Browne: *The History*; Bryceson and Pfaltzgraff: *Leprosy*, pp. 1-2.
18. Chaplin: *Diseases*, pp. 8-14.
19. Ibid., p. 9.
20. Masterman: *Hygiene*, pp. 17-18.
21. Morgenstern, Avraham, *Lepers and Leprosy in Jerusalem: the Establishment of the German Leper Homes in the 19th Century*, M.A. thesis submitted to the University of Haifa 2006, pp. 17-18. The authors wish to thank Mr. Morgenstern for furnishing his manuscript.
22. Schwake: *Hospitals*, p. 252.

23. Levy: *The History*, pp. 128-129.
24. Chaplin's letter of May 18, 1877 in the *Report of the Leper Home* of 1877, quoted in Morgenstern: *Lepers*, p. 31-32. More on the hospital see: Marx, Theodor, *Die Elendesten der Elenden im Heiligen Lande. Das Aussätzigen-Asyl 'Jesus-Hilfe' in Jerusalem* (Herrnhut, 1906).
25. *Report of the Leper Home* (1882), p. 3, quoted in Morgenstern: *Lepers*, p. 41.
26. Ibid. (1905), p. 5, quoted in Morgenstern: *Lepers*, p. 55.
27. Seidler, E. 'An historical survey of children's hospitals', in: L. Granshaw and R. Porter (eds.), *The Hospital in History* (London and New York, 1990), pp. 184-187.
28. Still, George Fredric, *The History of Paediatrics* (London, 1965), p. 422.
29. Seidler: *Historical*, p.184.
30. Ibid., pp.184, 186-188.
31. Ibid., pp.189-190.
32. This chapter based mainly on Schwake: *Die Entwicklung*, II, pp. 634-646; Nissan, Shemuel and Martin, Petra, 'Max Sandreczky: A Pediatric Surgeon in 19th-Century Jerusalem', *Journal of Pediatric Surgery*, 33 (1998), pp. 1187-1193.
33. Schwake mention the fact that Theodor Fliedner, founder of the Deaconesses hospital in Jerusalem, raised that idea in a letter before his death in October 1864. See: Schwake: *Die Entwicklung*, II, p. 634.
34. Nissan and Martin: 'Max Sandreczky', p. 1188.
35. Nissan, Shemuel and Martin, Petra, 'A proposal to Establish a Children Hospital in 19th Century Jerusalem: Dr. Max Sandreczky to the Grossherzog Friedrich Franz II.', *Cathedra*, 107 (2003), pp. 173-175 [Hebrew].
36. Nissan and Martin: 'A proposal', pp. 173-176.
37. Nissan and Martin: 'Max Sandreczky', pp. 1188-1190; Nissan and Martin: 'A proposal', pp. 177-180.
38. Nissan and Martin: 'Max Sandreczky', pp. 1188-1190.
39. Nissan and Martin: 'Max Sandreczky', pp. 1188-1190; Nissan and Martin: 'A proposal', pp. 171-17.
40. Meyerhof, Max, 'A Short History of Ophthalmia during the Egyptian campaigns of 1798-1801', *The British Journal of Ophthalmology* (1932), p. 129-152; Ullmann, Manfred, *Islamic Medicine* (Edinburgh, 1978), pp. 1-6; Shimkin, N., 'Trachoma in Palestine; its epidemiology and a review of measures for dealing with it', *British Journal of Ophthalmology* (1926), pp. 265-267.
41. Bedford, R. William and Holbeche, Richard, *The Hospital of the Order of St. John of Jerusalem* (London, 1902), pp. 149-152; King, Edwin, *The Knights of St. John in the British Realm* (London, 1967), p. 163. For more

about the hospital, see: Izhaki, Rika, 'The Ophthalmic Hospital of the Order of St. John (1882-1948)', *Cathedra,* 67 (1993), pp. 114-135 [Hebrew]; Schwake: *Die Entwicklung*, pp. 647-652; Levy: *The History*, pp. 137-141

42. In May 14, 1882 as an answer to the request from the Prince of Wales, the Queen of England declared the society as: "*The Grand Priory of England of the Venerable Order of the Hospital of St. John of Jerusalem*", see: King: *The Knights*, p. 163.
43. Mehmed Rauf Pasha (1838-1923).
44. Bedford and Holbeche: *The Hospital*, pp. 150-152.
45. *British Ophthalmic Hospital*, Report of the Committee for 1886, p. 3.
46. Bedford and Holbeche: *The Hospital*, pp. 154-155.
47. Ibid., pp. 150-152.
48. Levy: *The History*, p. 138.
49. Bedford and Holbeche: *The Hospital*, pp. 156-158.
50. Ibid., pp. 155-156.
51. Ibid., p. 158; Izhaki: 'The Ophthalmic', pp. 120-123.
52. Bedford and Holbeche: *The Hospital*, pp. 161-162.
53. King: *The Knights*, p. 167.
54. Izhaki: 'The Ophthalmic', p. 123.
55. On the Temple Society see: Carmel, Alex, *Die Siedlungen der württembergischen Templer in Palästina 1868 1918. Ihre lokalpolitischen und internationalen Probleme* (3rd ed.) (Stuttgart, 2000); Lange, Friedrich, *Geschichte des Tempel* (Stuttgart, 1899); Sauer, Paul, *The Holy Land Called: The Story of the Temple Society* (Melbourne, 1991); Perry, Yaron, Tempelgesellschaft (Deutscher Tempel), *Religion in Geschichte und Gegenwart (RGG*[4]*)*, (Tübingen, 2005), vol. 8, pp. 154-155.
56. On the American colony in Jaffa see: Holmes, Reed, *The Forerunners*, (Independence, Mo., 1981). On the German colony see: Eisler, Ejal Jakob, *Der deutsche Beitrag zum Aufstieg Jaffas 1850-1914. Zur Geschichte Palästinas im 19.Jahrhundert* (Wiesbaden, 1997).
57. *Die Warte des Tempels* (May 31, 1928), pp. 73-78.
58. On him see: Eisler, Ejal Jakob, *Peter Martin Metzler (1824-1907). Ein christlicher Missionar im Heiligen Land* (Haifa, 1999).
59. Eisler: *Metzler*, pp. 29-45.
60. On the hardship at the early days of Sarona, see: Glenk, Helmut, *From Desert Sands to Golden Oranges. The History of the German Templar Settlements of Sarona in Palestine 1871-1947* (Victoria – Canada, 2005), pp. 13-19.
61. *Die Warte* (May 31, 1928), pp. 73-78.
62. Rubitschung, Otto, *Das Deutsche Krankenhaus in Jaffa 1869 bis 1927*, Jerusalem [1928], pp. 16-17.

63. *Die Warte* (May 31, 1928), pp. 73-78.
64. Ibid.
65. Rubitschung: *Deutsche*, pp. 29-30. For more on the hospital see: Rubitschung, Otto, *Der Werdegang des deutschen Krankenhauses in Jaffa* (Jerusalem, 1927).
66. Wilkinson J., *The Coogate Doctors, The History of the Edinburgh Medical Missionary Society 1841-1991* (Edinburgh, 1991), pp. 43-45. On the Scottish mission see also: Marten, Michael, *Attempting to Bring the Gospel Home. Scottish Mission to Palestine 1839-1917* (London, 2006).
67. Wilkinson: *The Coogate*. pp. 43-45.
68. Mansur, A., *History of Nazareth* (Cairo, 1924). Bar-El, Yaron and Levy, Nissim, 'The Beginning of the Modern Medical Practice in Galilean Towns, 1860-1900', *Cathedra*, 54 (1989), pp. 96-106 [Hebrew].
69. Wilkinson: *The Coogate,* pp. 43-45.
70. Ziadat, Adel, 'Western Medicine in Palestine, 1860-1940: The Edinburgh Medical Missionary Society and its Hospital', *Canadian Bulletin of Medical History*, 10 (1993), pp. 269-279; Bishara, Nakhli. 'A Medical pioneer in Nazareth', *Korot*, 12 (1996-1997), pp. 124-136.
71. *Edinburgh Medical Missionary Society Quarterly Paper*, I (1871), pp. 132-133; Bishara: 'A Medical'.
72. Ziadat: 'Western'; Bishara: 'A Medical'. In 1867 Vartan treated two Germans of the Templar Society in their early attempts to settled in Palestine. See: Goren, Haim, 'The earliest Templar Settlement in the Holy Land', in: E. Schiller (ed.), *Zev Vilnay's Jubilee Volume* (Jerusalem, 1987), vol. 2, p. 272 [Hebrew].
73. Wilkinson: *The Coogate,* p. 44.
74. Ziadat: 'Western'.
75. Ibid.; Wilkinson: *The Coogate*, p. 44; Schwake: *Hospitals*, pp. 256-257.
76. Wilkinson, *The Coogate*, p. 44; *Edinburgh Medical*: XII (1909), pp. 114-115.
77. Bar-El and Levy: 'The Beginning'.
78. Ewing, W., 'Palestine Revisited after Eighteen Years', *The Missionary Records of the United Free Church of Scotland*, 7 (1912), p. 311.
79. *Edinburgh Medical*: XXVII (1899), pp. 368-370.
80. Ibid., LXII (1906), pp. 231-233.
81. Wilkinson: *The Coogate*, pp. 45-46.
82. Ibid., p. 47.
83. Livingstone, William Pringale, *A Galilee Doctor. Being a Sketch of the Career of Dr. D.W. Torrance of Tiberias* (London [1922]), pp. 57-58.
84. Bar-El and Levy: 'The Beginning', pp. 96-99.

85. Stuart, A. Moody, 'The Origin of the Mission', in: J. H. Wilson and J. Wells (eds.), *The Sea of Galilee Mission of the Free Church of Scotland* (Edinburgh and London, 1896), pp. 13-21.
86. Wilson, H., 'The Revival of the Original Proposal in 1883', in: Wilson and Wells: *Sea of Galilee*, pp. 25-29.
87. Livingstone: *A Galilee*, p. 23-24. More about his youth see: ibid., pp. 10-23. More about the hospital see: Marten, *Attempting*, pp. 63-84.
88. Wells, Torrance and Laidlaw in a letter from Jerusalem, April 8, 1884, in: *Report on the Conversion of the Jews* (of the Free Church of Scotland), 1884, p. 3-4.
89. Wells, J., 'The Deputation of 1884', in: Wilson and Wells: *Sea of Galilee*, pp. 30-39. On the 1839 expedition see: Bonar, Andrew and M'Cheyne, Robert Murray, *Narrative of a mission of inquiry to the Jews from the Church of Scotland in 1839* (Philadelphia, 1845).
90. Torrance, W. David, 'The Planting of the Mission in 1885', in: Wilson and Wells: *Sea of Galilee*, pp. 40-55.
91. Ibid.
92. Bar-El and Levy: 'The Beginning'.
93. Torrance: 'The Planting'.
94. Wilson, G., 'The History of the Hospital', in: Wilson and Wells: *Sea of Galilee*, pp. 56-83. See there also description in details of the "methods of work" e.g. the missionary as well medical work in the hospital.
95. *The Missionary Records of the United Free Church of Scotland*, VIII (1908), p. 460.
96. Muir, Ernest, 'Tiberias Hospital', *The Missionary Records of the United Free Church of Scotland*, 4 (1904), p.168.
97. Mirbach, Ernst, Freiherr von (ed.), *Das deutsche Kaiserpaar im Heiligen Lande im Herbst 1898* (Berlin, 1899), p. 26.
98. Schwake: *Hospitals*, pp. 241-244. On the hospital see also: Langlois, Claude, 'Les congrégations Françaises en Terre Sainte au XIX siècle' in: D. Trimbur and R. Aaronsohn (eds.), *De Bonaparte à Balfour - La France, l'Europe occidentale et la Palestine, 1799-1917*, collection "Mélanges" du CRFJ, vol. 3, (Paris, 2001), pp. 219-240.
99. Tobler: *Denkblätter*, pp. 403-404. Tobler suggested that the Catholic institution was founded to compete with the English mission hospital.
100. Schwake: *Hospitals*, pp. 241-244. Mendelssohn left Jerusalem to Constantinople were he died in 1854.
101. Ibid., pp. 241-244.
102. Shilony, Zvi, 'The Activity of the Comte de Piéllat in Palestine (1884-1925)', *Cathedra*, 72 (1994), pp. 63-90.
103. Ibid.

104. Schwake: *Hospitals*, p. 254
105. Caboga acquired this plot after he failed to buy the ruin of the medieval hospital of St. John. See more about it in: Stransky, Thomas, 'The Austrian Hospital at Tantur (1869-1918)', in: M. Wrba (ed.), *Austrian Presence in the Holy Land in the 19th and Early 20th Century* (Tel Aviv, 1996). pp. 98-101.
106. Stransky: 'The Austrian', pp. 101-106.
107. Schwacke, Norbert, 'The Austrian Hospital in Nazareth', in: M. Wrba (ed.), *Austrian Presence in the Holy Land in the 19th and Early 20th Century* (Tel Aviv, 1996), p. 82; Stransky: 'The Austrian', p. 107.
108. Stransky: 'The Austrian', p. 111.
109. Ibid., pp. 111-112.
110. Schwake: *Hospitals*, p. 255.
111. Eliav, Mordechai, *Under Imperial Austrian Protection: selected documents from the archives of the Austrian consulate in Jerusalem (1849-1917)* (Jerusalem, 1985), p. 290, file: Jer. I/14 ad No. 16 [Hebrew].
112. Stransky: 'The Austrian', p. 115.
113. Ibid., pp. 83-84.
114. Schwake: *Hospitals*, pp. 255-256; 1966a, pp. 86-88.
115. Ibid., p. 256; 1996a, p. 86.
116. Rabba, Yoel, *Erets Israel in the Descriptions of Russian pilgrims* (Jerusalem, 1987), pp. 12-13 [Hebrew]. On the Russian presence in Palestine see: Hopwood, Derek, *The Russian Presence in Syria and Palestine 1834-1914. Church and Politics in the Near East* (Oxford, 1969); Stavrou, Theofanis George, *Russian Interests in Palestine 1882-1914. A study of Religious and Educational Enterprise* (Thessaloniki, 1963).
117. On the hospital see mainly in: Schwake: *Die Entwicklung*, pp. 419-426.
118. Wolff, Philipp, 'Rückblicke auf die jüngste Geschichte Jerusalems von Jahre 1856 bis 1866', *Sieben Artikel über Jerusalem aus den Jahren 1859 bis 1869* (Stuttgart, 1869), pp. 49-58, quoted in Schwake: *Die Entwicklung*, p. 420; Neuman, Bernard, *Die Heilige Stadt und deren Bewohner* (Hamburg, 1877), p. 311.
119. Luntz, Abraham Moses, *Luach Eretz Israel* (Jerusalem, 1887), p. 89 [Hebrew].
120. Schwake: *Hospitals*, p. 421; Levy: *The History*, p. 115.
121. Tsibkin, Vladimir, 'The Palestinian Imperial Pravoslavic Society (1882-1914)', *Cathedra*, 46 (1987), pp. 83-84 [Hebrew]; Habibi, Eliyahu and Lahav, Meir, 'The history of the Russian hospital in Jerusalem', *Ariel*, 100-101 (1994), pp. 67-69 [Hebrew]; Levy: *The History*, pp. 115-117.
122. Tsibkin: 'The Palestinian', p. 83.
123. Schwake: *Hospitals*, pp. 253; Levy: *The History*, p. 117.

124. Greenberg: *The Turkish.*
125. Cuinet, Vital, *Syrie, Liban et Palestine: Géographie administrative, statistique, descriptive et raisonnée* (Paris, 1896), II, pp. 560-561.
126. Cuinet: *Syrie*, II, pp. 553-554.
127. Greenberg: 'The Turkish', pp. 57-58.
128. Ibid., pp.59-61.
129. *Allgemeine Zeitung des Judenthums* No. 39, September 24, 1842. More about this hospital see: Morgenstern, Avraham, 'The First Jewish Hospital in Jerusalem', *Cathedra*, 33 (1984), pp. 107-124; Levy: *The History*, pp. 43-51; Schwake: *Die Entwicklung*, I, pp. 193-244.
130. Morgenstern: 'The First'.
131. Eliav, Mordechai, *Love of Zion and Men of Hod, German Jewry and the settlement of Eretz-Irael in the 19th century* (Tel Aviv, 1970), pp. 287-290.
132. *Allgemeine Zeitung des Judenthums*, No. 3, January 2, 1843.
133. Gragewski: *In Memory*, pp. 3-4.
134. *Jewish Intelligence* (August 1843), p. 287.
135. Count of Lantivy, the French Consul in Jerusalem, who sent a letter on October 6, 1844, to James de Rothschild in Paris, accusing Fränkel of exacting high fees for the drugs he distributed to his patients and of treating preferentially young and beautiful women, whereas the old and unsightly were left unattended. The urge not to support the establishment of a hospital, based on these accusations served its purpose; the money never reached Philippson. See: Kottek, Samuel and Schwake, Norbert, 'The first Jewish Hospital in Jerusalem', *Medicine's Geographic Heritage*, 4 (1988), pp. 3-9.
136. Eliav: *Love*, pp. 287-290.
137. *Allgemeine Zeitung des Judenthums* No. 10, March 4, 1844.
138. *Jewish Intelligence* (March 1845), p. 89.
139. Tobler: *Denkblätter*, pp. 410-411.
140. Fliender, Theodor, *Reisen in das heilige Land* (Düsseldorf, 1858), p. 180.
141. Tobler, Titus, Dritte Wanderung nach Palästina (Gotha, 1859), p. 324.
142. Levy: *The History*, pp. 43-51; Schwake: *Die Entwicklung*, vol. 1, pp. 193-244.
143. Loewe, Louis, *Diaries of Sir Moses Montefiore* (London, 1890), vol. 2, pp. 24-25; Kottek and Schwake: *'The first'*; Kass, Amalie, 'Sir Moses Montefiore and medical philanthropy in the Holy Land', in: M. Wasserman and S. Kottek (eds.), *Health and Diseases in the Holy Land* (New York, 1996), p. 219.
144. While negotiating with the Touro party over the exact plans for using the money, and before Montefiore took his forth journey to Palestine, the Rothschilds entered the scene again. As a quick response to the

harsh situation in Jerusalem, the French branch of the family sent a delegate who committed the Rothschild fund for the establishment of a hospital.

145. Loewe: *Diaries*, vol. 2, p. 38.
146. Kass: 'Sir Moses', p. 220.
147. Schischa, A., 'The Saga of 1855: A Study in Depth', in: S. and V.D. Lipman, *Century of Moses Montefiore* (Oxford, 1985), p. 292, cited in Kass: 'Sir Moses', p. 221.
148. Loewe: *Diaries*, vol. 2, p. 42.
149. Ibid., pp. 52-53; Kass: 'Sir Moses', pp. 219, 222.
150. The detailed report was written by Frankel, Ludwig August, *Nach Jerusalem* (Leipzig, 1858), pp. 116-118. Cited in Shwake: *Die Entwicklung*, pp. 232-233.
151. Kass: 'Sir Moses', p. 225.
152. Schischa: 'The Saga', p. 279; Kass: 'Sir Moses', p. 220.
153. Dr Edward Macgowan, attending without being invited, reported on July 1854 that the inauguration of the hospital took place with as imposing a ceremony as circumstances could permit. 'The building appropriated for the hospital is a new and handsome erection which had been destined for a school'. See: *Jewish Intelligence* (September 1854), p. 284.
154. About him see in his book: Neuman: *Die Heilige*.
155. Kottek and Schwake: 'The first'.
156. Pizzamano to Constantinople, 2.2.1860, F28/3. S. 37-38 in: Eliav: *Under*, p. 122.
157. Alfonse de Rothschild to Pizzamano, Paris February 5, 1857, Jer. II/39 XL III in: Eliav: *Under*, no. 29, pp. 106-107.
158. Pizzamano to Prokesch-Osten, Jerusalem 2.2.1860, F28/3 in: Eliav: *Under*, no. 37, pp. 122-124.
159. Schwake: *Hospitals*, pp. 245-246.
160. Kwiatkowski to Rothschild, 7.8.1893, Jer. II/75. No. 724, in: Eliav: *Under*, pp. 250-252.
161. Leopold Walcher von Moltheim (1823-1911) the Austrian Consul to Constantinople, 25.10.1865, Jer. II/47, No. 9, in: Eliav: *Under*, pp. 137-138.
162. Eliav: *Under*, p.137.
163. Freidin: 'Bikur Holim', pp. 117-140.
164. Schwake: *Hospitals*, pp. 247.
165. Rechberg to Franz Josef, F28/5, in: Eliav: *Under*, no. 41, pp. 129-130.
166. Hanauer, James Edward, *Walks In and Around Jerusalem* (London, 1926), p. 27.
167. Schwake: *Hospitals*, pp. 247.

168. Philipsborn to Baron Karl Victor von Alten (1800-1871), 16.1.1871, in: Eliav, Mordechai, *The Jews of Palestine in the German Policy. Selected Documents from the Archives of the German Consulates in Jerusalem 1842-1914* (Tel Aviv, 1973), p. 30, No. 35.
169. Schwake: *Hospitals*, pp. 247-248.
170. Einsler to the German Consulate in Jerusalem, 3.10.1898, in Eliav: *The Jews*, No. 170, p. 138.
171. Solomon, Pinnes and Levi to the Austrian Home Office, 15.11.1905, F11/94, No. 1833, in: Eliav: *Under*, no. 140, pp. 311-312.
172. Series of letters in Record Group 67 (Archives of the German Consulate in Jerusalem) in the Israel State Archive, quoted in: Eliav: *The Jews*, pp. 106-110. Reitz to Raouf Pasha, 28.8.1884; Copy of the Governor's reply, 3.9.1884; Reitz to Radowitz, 5.11.1884; Lehmann to Reitz, 13.11.1884; Reitz to Lehmann, 19.1.1885; Radowitz to Reitz, 26.2.1885.
173. Schwake: Hospitals, pp. 250; Porush, E., *Sha'are Tsedek: To the History of the Hospital and its First Director* (Jerusalem, 1952), pp. 9-13 [Hebrew].
174. Radolin to Tischendorf. 17.7.1893, in: Eliav: *The Jews*, No 154, p. 125.
175. On Frutiger and his contribution to the development of the Jewish settlements in Jerusalem, see: Carmel: 'Der Bankier'.
176. Eliav: *Love*, p. 295.
177. Porush: *Sha'are Tsedek*, pp. 18-25.
178. Wallach to Schmidt, 8.8.1902 in: Eliav: *The Jews*, No. 176, p. 145-146.
179. Levy: *The History*, p. 75-76.
180. Qashani, Reuben, *Misgav Ladach, General Hospital in Jerusalem: 120 Years Anniversary* (Jerusalem, 1976), pp. 23-26; Schwake: *Hospitals*, pp. 245-246.
181. Levy: *The History*, p. 75.
182. Ibid., p. 76.
183. Schwake: *Hospitals*, pp. 245-246; Levy: *The History*, p. 75-77.
184. Levy: *The History*, p. 78.
185. Schwake: *Hospitals*, p. 246.

Postscript and Appendixes

1. Wheeler and Masterman to Dickson, Jerusalem November 13, 1900, FO 195/2084, in: Eliav, Mordechai, *Britain and the Holy Land 1838-1914: Selected Documents from the British Consulate in Jerusalem* (Jerusalem, 1997), no. 85, pp. 293-295.
2. Rooker, J., *Half-an-Hour in a… Jerusalem Dispensary*, A pamphlet published by the London Jews Society [1907], pp. 3-14, in: St. Albans.
3. ITAC, Medical Diaries, pp. 226-237.

4. Ibid., pp.1-8.
5. Seidler, '*An historical*', pp. 181-197, 182-184.
6. Sticker, Anna D., *Theodor Fliedner and Nursing* (Kaiserswerth 1972).
7. Nightingale: *The Institution*, pp. 5-34.
8. ITAC, Medical diaries, pp. 381-383, 386.

BIBLIOGRAPHY

Journals and periodicals

Allgemeine Zeitung des Judenthums, Leipzig (1837-1922)

Bericht über die Diakonissen-Stationen im Morgenlande, Kaiserswerth (1851-1899)

Die Warte des Tempels, Stuttgart (1845-)

Edinburgh Medical Missionary Society Quarterly Paper

Jewish Expositor and the Friends of Israel, containing monthly communication respecting the Jews, and the proceedings of the London Society, London (1816-1829)

Jewish Intelligence - Monthly Account of the Proceedings of the London Society for Promoting Christianity Amongst the Jews, London (1835-1892)

Jewish Missionary Intelligence - the Monthly Record of the London Society for Promoting Christianity Amongst the Jews, London (1893-1962)

Missionary Herald, American Board of Foreign Missions, Boston (1831-1934)

Missionary Records of the United Free Church of Scotland

Palestine Exploration Quarterly, London (1869-)

Report of the London Society for Promoting Christianity Amongst the Jews, London (1809-1910)

Report on the Conversion of the Jews (of the Free Church of Scotland)

Times, London (1875-)

Books and Articles

Abeken, Heinrich, *The Protestant Bishopric in Jerusalem: Its Origin and Progress. From the Official Documents Published by Command of His Majesty the King of Prussia and from other Authentic Sources* (London, 1847).

Amar, Zohar and Lev, Efraim, 'An Early Glimpse at Western Medicine in Jerusalem 1700-1840: The Case of the Jews and the Franciscans Medical Activity', *Vesalius*, 11(2) (2005), pp. 81-87.

Amar, Zohar and Lev, Efraim, 'Traditional Medicinal Substances in Jerusalem According to Titus Tobler', *Harefuah*, 138 (2000), pp. 604-607.

Amar, Zohar and Lev, Efraim, *Physicians, Drugs and Remedies in Jerusalem from the 10th to the 18th Centuries* (Tel-Aviv, 2000) [Hebrew].

Amar, Zohar, 'The Export of Theriac from the Land of Israel and its Uses in the Middle Ages', *Korot*, 12 (1996-1997), pp. 16-29 [Hebrew].

Amar, Zohar, 'The preservation of sacred healing sites in Jerusalem', in: *Judea and Samaria Research Studies – Proceedings of the Seventh Conference* (1997), pp. 207-222 [Hebrew].

Amar, Zohar, *The history of medicine in Jerusalem* (Oxford, 2002).

Anno., 'Obituary Notice, Masterman, Ernest William Gurney', *Palestine Exploration Quarterly*, 75 (1943), pp. 70-73.

Anon., 'Obituary Notice, Dr Percy d'Erf Wheeler, F.R.C.S.', *Palestine Exploration Quarterly*, 77 (1945), pp. 54-55.

Arce, Alonso, *Miscelanea de Tierra Santa*, 2 vols. (Jerusalem, 1950).

Baedeker, Karl (ed.), *Jerusalem and its Surroundings* (Leipsic, 1876).

Bagatti, Battista, 'Father Anthony Manzazi of Cuna (1650–1729), of Inventor the Balm of Jerusalem', *Franciscan Studies*, 6 (1946), pp. 250–361.

Bannurah, Thomas, *History of Bethlehem, Beit Jala and Beit Sachour* (Jerusalem, 1982) [Arabic].

Bar El, Yaron and Levy, Nissim, 'The Beginning of the Modern Medical Practice in Galilean Towns, 1860-1900', *Cathedra*, 54 (1989), pp. 96-106 [Hebrew].

Bedford, R. William and Holbeche, Richard, *The Hospital of the Order of St. John of Jerusalem* (London, 1902).

Ben Arieh, Yehoshua, 'The Landscape of Palestine on the Eve of the Zionist Colonization', in: I. Kolatt (ed.) *The History of the Jewish Community in Eretz-Israel since 1882: The Ottoman Period* (Jerusalem, 1989), pp. 75-141 [Hebrew].

Ben Arieh, Yehoshua, *Jerusalem in the 19th century, the Old City* (Jerusalem, 1984).

Ben Arzi, Yossi, 'Johannes Zeller – a missionary to Nazareth and the Holy Land', *Cathedra*, 50 (1989), 73-97 [Hebrew].

Ben Maimon, Moses, *On Asthma*, in: S. Muntner (ed.) (Jerusalem, 1965) [Hebrew].

Benayahu, Meir, *Essays on Medicine by Rabbi Rephael Mordecai Malki* (Jerusalem, 1988) [Hebrew]

Benayahu, Meir, *Medical Works of Rabbi Rafael Mordecai Malki* (Jerusalem, 1985) [Hebrew].

Bishara, Nakhli, 'A Medical pioneer in Nazareth', *Korot*, 12 (1996-1997), pp. 124-136.

Bonar, Andrew and M'Cheyne, Robert Murray, *Narrative of a Mission of Inquiry to the Jews from the Church of Scotland in 1839* (Philadelphia, 1845).

British Pharmacopoeia (London, 1858).

Brown, Frank and Masterman, Ernest William Gurney, 'Two cases of strangulated umbilical hernia', *Lancet*, I (1916), p. 1217.

Browne, Stanley George, 'The History of Leprosy', in: R.C. Hastings (ed), *Leprosy* (Edinburgh, London and New York, 1985).

Bruenn, W. and Goldberg, L., 'Die Malaria Jerusalems und ihre Bekämpfung', *Zeitschrift für Hygiene und Infektionskrankheiten*, 75 (1913), pp. 209-235.

Bryceson, Aanthony and Pfaltzgraff, E. Roy, *Leprosy* (Edinburgh, London and New York, 1979).

Buchan, A., 'Remarks on the Climate of Jerusalem, from Observations made by Dr Thomas Chaplin for three years and four months, beginning November 1, 1863, and ending February 28, 1867', *Palestine Exploration Quarterly*, 3 (1872), pp. 19-30.

Bunsen, Frances, *A Memoir of Baron Bunsen, Drawn Chiefly from Family Papers by his Widow Frances Bunsen*, 2 vols. (2nd ed.) (London, 1869).

Carmel, Alex, 'Activities of the European Powers in Palestine 1799-1914', *Asian and African Studies*, 19 (1985), pp. 43-92.

Carmel, Alex, 'Der Bankier Johannes Frutiger und seine Zeitgenossen. Entstehen und Untergang der Basler Firma C.F. Spittler in Jerusalem', *Pietismus und Neuzeit*, 11 (1985), pp. 139-158.

Carmel, Alex, 'Der Missionar Theodor Fliedner als Pionier deutscher Palästina-Arbeit', in: G. Walter (ed.), *Jahrbuch des Instituts für Deutsche Geschichte* (Tel Aviv, 1985), vol. XIV, pp. 191-220.

Carmel, Alex, 'Jerusalem muss unser werden. Titus Tobler und der 'Christenstaat'', in: H. Haumann (ed.), *Der Traum von Israel* (Weinheim, 1998).

Carmel, Alex, 'Wie es zu Conrad Schicks Sendung nach Jerusalem kam', in: *Zeitschrift des Deutschen Palästina-Vereins (ZDPV)*, 99 (1983), pp. 204-218

Carmel, Alex, *Die Siedlungen der württembergischen Templer in Palästina 1868-1918. Ihre lokalpolitischen und internationalen Probleme* (3rd ed.) (Stuttgart, 2000).

Carmel, Alex, *Palästina-Chronik, 1853 bis 1882* (Ulm, 1978).

Chaplin, Thomas, 'An Ancient Hebrew Weight from Samaria', *Palestine Exploration Quarterly*, 22 (1890), pp. 267-268.

Chaplin, Thomas, 'Beth Habbechereh, or the Chosen House', *Palestine Exploration Quarterly*, 17 (1885), pp. 29-56, 140-147, 184-196.

Chaplin, Thomas, 'Gihon', *Palestine Exploration Quarterly*, 22 (1890), pp. 124-125, 331.

Chaplin, Thomas, 'Greek Inscription on A Stone Found at Samaria, now in Possession of Yakoob Esh Shellaby', *Palestine Exploration Quarterly*, 3 (1871), p. 134.

Chaplin, Thomas, 'Letter from Dr. Chaplin', *Palestine Exploration Quarterly*, 3 (1871), pp. 101-103.

Chaplin, Thomas, 'Letter from Thomas Chaplin', *Palestine Exploration Quarterly*, 26 (1894), pp. 225.

Chaplin, Thomas, 'Letters from Dr. Chaplin', *Palestine Exploration Quarterly*, 5 (1873), pp. 155-157.

Chaplin, Thomas, 'Modern Palestine', *The Churchman*, (October-November 1887), pp. 43-53, 85-95.

Chaplin, Thomas, 'Note on M. Ganneau's Paper, "The Arab in Palestine"', *Palestine Exploration Quarterly*, 8 (1876), pp. 8-9.

Chaplin, Thomas, 'Observations on the Climate of Jerusalem', *Palestine Exploration Quarterly*, 15 (1883), pp. 8-40.

Chaplin, Thomas, 'On Malarial Typhoid Fever', *Lancet*, 22 (1885), pp. 518-520.

Chaplin, Thomas, 'On the Case of Leuce', *Lancet*, 6 (1868), p. 656.

Chaplin, Thomas, 'Some Jerusalem Notes', *Palestine Exploration Quarterly*, 21 (1889), pp. 9-11.

Chaplin, Thomas, 'The Climate of Jerusalem', *Palestine Exploration Quarterly*, 5 (1873), pp. 39.

Chaplin, Thomas, 'The Fevers of Jerusalem', *Lancet*, 2 (1864), pp. 236-238, 256-269, 289-291.

Chaplin, Thomas, 'The Site of Ebenezer', *Palestine Exploration Quarterly*, 20 (1888), pp. 263-265.

Chaplin, Thomas, 'The Stone of Foundation and the Site of the Temple', *Palestine Exploration Quarterly*, 8 (1876), pp. 22-28.

Chaplin, Thomas, 'The Visit of David the Reubenite to Hebron and Jerusalem in A.D. 1523', *Palestine Exploration Quarterly*, 29 (1897), pp. 44-53.

Chaplin, Thomas, 'Tomb at Jerusalem', *Palestine Exploration Quarterly*, 8 (1876), pp. 61-62.

Chaplin, Thomas, 'Yoma, or the Day of Atonement', *Palestine Exploration Quarterly*, 17 (1885), pp. 197-207, 286-293.

Chaplin, Thomas, *On Some Diseases Mentioned in the Bible* (London, 1902).

Circlli, A., *Gli Annali di Terra Sante* (Karachi, 1918).

Cohn Erich, 'The Deaconesses of Kaiserswerth', *Women in Jerusalem* (unpublished manuscript: Second Draught (July 1994).

Corey, W. Muriel, *From Rabbi to Bishop, the Biography of the Right Reverend Michael Solomon Alexander, Bishop in Jerusalem* (London, [1956]).

Craft, T.M. and Upton, P.M., *Key Topics in Anaesthesia* (Oxford, 1992),

Crombie, Kelvin, *For the Love of Zion. Christian Witness and the Restoration of Israel* (London 1991).

Cropper, John, 'The geographical distribution of anopheles and Malarial fever in Upper Palestine', *Journal of Hygiene*, 2 (1902), pp. 47-57.

Cropper, John, 'The Malaria fevers of Jerusalem and their prevention', *Journal of Hygiene*, 5 (1905), pp. 460-466

Cuinet, Vital, *Syrie, Liban et Palestine: Géographie administrative, statistique, descriptive et raisonnée* (Paris, 1896).

Cumming, James Elder, 'Notes on Medical Mission', *The Church of Scotland Home and Foreign Missionary Record*, 1 (October 1879), pp. 492-494.

Cunningham, Andrew and Williams, Perry (eds.), *The Laboratory Revolution in Medicine* (Cambridge, 1992). pp. 1-13.

Duncan, Andrew, *The Edinburgh New Dispensatory* (Edinburgh, 1804).

Eisler, Ejal Jakob, *Der deutsche Beitrag zum Aufstieg Jaffas 1850-1914. Zur Geschichte Palästinas im 19.Jahrhundert* (Wiesbaden, 1997).

Eisler, Ejal Jakob, *Peter Martin Metzler (1824-1907). Ein christlicher Missionar im Heiligen Land* (Haifa, 1999).

Eliav, Mordechai, *Britain and the Holy Land 1838-1914: Selected Documents from the British Consulate in Jerusalem* (Jerusalem, 1997).

Eliav, Mordechai, *Love of Zion and Men of Hod, German Jewry and the settlement of Eretz-Irael in the 19th century* (Tel Aviv, 1970) [Hebrew].

Eliav, Mordechai, *The Jews of Palestine in the German Policy. Selected Documents from the Archives of the German Consulates in Jerusalem 1842-1914* (Tel Aviv, 1973) [Hebrew and German].

Eliav, Mordechai, *Under Imperial Austrian Protection: selected documents from the archives of the Austrian Consulate in Jerusalem (1849-1917)* (Jerusalem, 1985) [Hebrew].

Encyclopedia Biblica (Jerusalem, 1956).

Ewing, W., 'Palestine Revisited after Eighteen Years', *The Missionary Records of the United Free Church of Scotland*, 7 (1912), p. 311.

Fliedner, Georg, *Theodor Fliedner. Sein Leben und Wirken*, 2 vols. (Kaiserswerth, 1908, 1910).

Fliender, Theodor, *Reisen in das heilige Land* (Düsseldorf, 1858).

Frankel, Ludwig August, *Nach Jerusalem* (Leipzig, 1858).

Freidin, Israel, 'Bikur Holim Perushim in Jerusalem – From Society to Hospital', *Cathedra*, 23 (1983), pp. 117-140 [Hebrew].

Gidney, William Thomas, *History of the London Society for Promoting Christianity amongst the Jews* (London, 1908).

Glenk, Helmut, *From Desert Sands to Golden Oranges. The History of the German Templar Settlement of Sarona in Palestine 1871-1947* (Victoria – Canada, 2005).

Goldreich, Yair, *The Climate of Israel: Observations, Research and Applications* (New York, 2003).

Goren H. (ed.), *Conrad Schick. For the Sake of Jerusalem*, in: *Ariel* series, 130-131) (Jerusalem 1998) [Hebrew].

Goren, Haim, 'The earliest Templar Settlement in the Holy Land', in: E. Schiller (ed.) *Zev Vilnay's Jubilee Volume*, 2 vols. (Jerusalem, 1987) [Hebrew].

Grajewski, Pinchas Ben Zion, 'Letter from Montefiore to the Rabbis of the Jewish Community', in: P. B-Z., Grajewski (ed.), *In Memory of the First Zionists* (Jerusalem, 1928),

Grajewski, Pinchas Ben Zion, *In Memory of the First Zionists*, (Jerusalem,1928).

Grajewski, Pinchas Ben Zion, *The Struggle of the Jews against the Mission from 1824 till our Times* (Jerusalem, 1935).

Gran, Peter, 'Medical Pluralism in Arab and Egyptian History: An Overview of Class Structures and Philosophies of the Main Phases', *Social Science and Medicine*, 13 (1979), pp. 339-348.

Granshaw, Lindsay, 'Fame and fortune by means of bricks and mortar: the medical profession and specialist hospitals in Britain, 1800-1948', in: L. Granshaw and R. Porter (eds.), *The Hospital in History* (London and New York, 1990), pp. 199-200.

Greenberg, Zalman, 'The Earliest Medical Article from the Holy Land', *Harefua*, 124(9) (1993), pp. 581-588 [Hebrew].

Greenberg, Zalman, 'The Turkish Municipal Hospital in Jerusalem and its Director Dr. Photios Efklides', in: N. Sari, A.H. Bayat, Y. Ulman and M. Isin (eds.), *Proceedings of the 38th International Congress on the History of Medicine*, Ankara 2005, pp. 1417-1420.

Greenberg, Zalman, 'The Turkish Municipal Hospital in Jerusalem', *Cathedra*, 78 (1995), pp. 49-64 [Hebrew].

Guérin, Victor, *Jerusalem: son histoire, sa description, ses établissements religieux* (Paris, 1889).

Habibi, Eliyahu and Lahav, Meir, 'The history of the Russian hospital in Jerusalem', *Ariel* 100-101(1994), pp. 65-75 [Hebrew].

Hanauer, James Edward and Masterman, Ernest William Gurney, *Cook's Hand Book for Palestine and Syria* (London, 1907).

Hanauer, James Edward, *Walks In and around Jerusalem* (London, 1926).

Hansen, A. Gerald, 'On the Etiology of Leprosy', *Chirurgical Review*, 55 (1875), pp. 459-489.

Harrison, Gordon, *Mosquitoes, Malaria and Man: A History of the Hostilities Since 1880* (New York, 1978), pp. 10, 33, 102-104.

Hartum, Menachem Emanuele and David, Abraham, *From Italy to Jerusalem: Letters of Rabbi Obadiah mi-Bartenura* (Jerusalem, 1997) [Hebrew].

Hasselquist, Friedrich, *Voyages and Travels in the Levant* (London, 1866),

Hechler, William Henry, *The Jerusalem Bishopric,1841. Documents Chiefly Reprinted from a Copy of the Original German Account, 'Das Evangelische Bisthum in Jerusalem'. Geschichtliche Darlegung mit Urkunden* (Berlin, 1842; London, 1883).

Heim, Heinrich Jakob, *Dr. Titus Tobler, der Palästinafahrer, ein appenzellisches Lebensbild* (Zürich und Torgen, 1879).

Holmes, Reed, *The Forerunners* (Independence, Mo., 1981).

Hopwood, Derek, *The Russian Presence in Syria and Palestine 1834-1914. Church and Politics in the Near East* (Oxford, 1969).

Horn, Elzar, 'Ichnographiae Monumentorum Terrae Sanctae', in: E. Hoade and B. Bagatti (eds.), *Studium Biblicum Franciscanum*, No. 15 (Jerusalem, 1962).

Hyamson, Albert Montefiore, *The British Consulate in Jerusalem in Relation to the Jews of Palestine 1838-1914*, 2 vols. (London, 1939).

Izhaki, Rivka, 'The Ophthalmic Hospital of the Order of St. John (1882-1948)', *Cathedra*, 67 (1993), pp. 114-135 [Hebrew].

Kark, Ruth, 'Millenarism and Agricultural Settlement in the Holy Land in the Nineteenth Century', *Journal of Historical Geography*, 9 (1983), pp. 46-62.

Kass, Amalie, 'Sir Moses Montefiore and medical philanthropy in the Holy Land', in: M. Wasserman and S. Kottek (eds.), *Health and Diseases in the Holy Land* (New York, 1996), pp. 207-230.

Kass, Amalie, 'Western Medicine in Nineteenth-Century Jerusalem', *Journal of the History of Medicine and Allied Sciences*, 44 (1989), pp. 447-461.

King, Edwin, *The Knights of St. John in the British Realm* (London, 1967).

Kloner, Amos and Zissu, Boaz, *The Necropolis of Jerusalem in the Second Temple Period* (Jerusalem, 2003) [Hebrew].

Kottek, Samuel and Schwake, Norbert, 'The first Jewish Hospital in Jerusalem', *Medicine's Geographic Heritage*, 4 (1988), pp. 3-9.

Lange, Friedrich, *Geschichte des Tempels* (Stuttgart, 1899).

Langlois, Claude, 'Les congrégations Françaises en Terre Sainte au XIX siècle' in: D. Trimbur and R. Aronsohn (eds.), *De Bonaparte à Balfour - La France, l'Europe occidentale et la Palestine,1799-1917*, collection 'Mélanges' du CRFJ, vol. 3, (Paris, 2001).

Lev, Efraim and Amar, Zohar, 'Ethnopharmacological Survey of Traditional Drugs Sold in Israel at the End of the 20th Century', *Journal of Ethnopharmacology*, 72 (2000), pp. 191-205.

Lev, Efraim and Amar, Zohar, 'The End of the Traditional Medicine in Jerusalem According to the Swiss Physician Titus Tobler (1806-1877)', *Canadian Bulletin for the History of Medicine*, 21 (2004), pp. 159-180.

Lev, Efraim and Perry, Yaron, 'Dr Edward Macgowan, a Long-Term Pioneer Physician in Mid-Nineteenth Century Jerusalem: Founder and Director of the First Modern Hospital in Palestine', *Journal of Medical Biography* (in press).

Lev, Efraim and Perry, Yaron, 'Dr Thomas Chaplin, Scientist and Scholar in Nineteenth-Century Palestine', *Palestine Exploration Quarterly*, 136 (2004), pp. 151-162.

Lev, Efraim and Perry, Yaron, 'The 1857 Inventory of Materia Medica of the British Hospital in Jerusalem', *Pharmaceutical Historian*, 32 (2002), pp. 40-45.

Lev, Efraim, 'Healing with Animals (Zootherapy) from Practical Medieval Medicine to Present-day Traditional Medicine in the Levant', *Journal of Ethnopharmacology*, 85 (2003), pp. 107-118.

Lev, Efraim, 'Healing with Animals in the Levant from 10th to 18th century', *Journal of Etnobiology and Ethnomedicine*, 2(11) (2006), pp. 1-11.

Lev, Efraim, 'Medical Materials in Jerusalem from the 10th to the 18th Centuries' in: Z. Amar, E. Lev and J. Schwartz (eds.),

Medicine in Jerusalem Throughout the Ages (Tel Aviv, 1999), pp. 51-78 [Hebrew].

Lev, Efraim, 'Medicinal Exploitation of Inorganic Substances in the Levant in the Medieval and Early Ottoman Periods', *Adler Museum Bulletin*, 28 (2002), pp. 11-16.

Lev, Efraim, 'Reconstructed materia medica of the Medieval and Ottoman al-Sham', *Journal of Ethnopharmacology*, 80 (2002), pp. 167-179.

Lev, Efraim, 'The Doctrine of Signature in the Medieval and Ottoman Levant', Vesalius, 8 (2002), pp. 1-10.

Lev, Efraim, *Medicinal Substances in Jerusalem from Early Times to Present Day*, (Oxford, 2003).

Lev, Efraim, *Medicinal Substances of the Medieval Levant* (Tel-Aviv, 2002) [Hebrew].

Levy, Nissim, *The History of Medicine in the Holy Land: 1799-1848* (Tel-Aviv, 1998) [Hebrew].

Lewis A. William, *A Complete Dictionary of the Whole Materia Medica* (London, 1810).

Livingstone, William Pringale, *A Galilee Doctor. Being a Sketch of the Career of Dr. D.W. Torrance of Tiberias* (London, [1922]).

Loewe, Louis, *Diaries of Sir Moses Montefiore* (London, 1890),

Lowe, J., *Jubillee Memorial* (Edinburgh, 1892).

Lückhoff, Martin, *Anglikaner und Protestanten im Heiligen Land* (Wiesbaden, 1998).

Luntz, Avraham Moses, *Jerusalem* (Jerusalem, 1889) [Hebrew].

Luntz, Avraham Moses, *Luach Eretz Israel* (Jerusalem, 1887) [Hebrew].

Macalister, Robert Alexander Stewart and Masterman, Ernest William Gurney, 'Occasional papers on the modern inhabitants of Palestine', *Palestine Exploration Quarterly*, 38 (1906), pp. 33-50, 110-114, 223-225, 286-291.

Macalister, Robert Alexander Stewart and Masterman, Ernest William Gurney, 'Diary of a visit to Safed', *Palestine Exploration Quarterly*, 39 (1907), pp. 91-130.

Mansur, A., *History of Nazareth* (Cairo, 1924).

Marten, Michael, *Attempting to Bring the Gospel Home. Scottish Mission to Palestine 1839-1917* (London, 2006).

Marx, Theodor, *Die Elendesten der Elenden im Heiligen Lande. Das Aussätzigen-Asyl 'Jesus-Hilfe' in Jerusalem* (Herrnhut, 1906).

Masterman, Ernest William Gurney, 'A case of death from diabetic coma after appendicectomy under local anaesthesia', *St. Bartholomew's Hospital Journal*, 21 (1913-14), p. 7.

Masterman, Ernest William Gurney, 'A case of successful caesarean section for eclampsia', *British Medical Journal*, II (1918), p. 342

Masterman, Ernest William Gurney, 'A Greek inscription from a column at Damascus', *Palestine Exploration Quarterly*, 28 (1896), pp. 340-341.

Masterman, Ernest William Gurney, 'A Greek inscription from the Grand Mosque, Damascus', *Palestine Exploration Quarterly*, 28 (1896), pp. 224-225.

Masterman, Ernest William Gurney, 'A smallpox epidemic in Jerusalem', *St. Bartholomew's Hospital Journal* (November 1900), pp. 19-21.

Masterman, Ernest William Gurney, 'Chephirah of Benjamin', *Palestine Exploration Quarterly*, 39 (1907), pp. 64-65.

Masterman, Ernest William Gurney, 'Ein El Feshkhah, El-Hajar El-Asbah and Khurbat Kumran', *Palestine Exploration Quarterly*, 34 (1902), pp. 297-299.

Masterman, Ernest William Gurney, 'Haemoglobinuric fever in Syria, and some notes on the occurrence of the disease in Palestine', *British Medical Journal*, 1 (1906), pp. 314-315.

Masterman, Ernest William Gurney, 'Hirudinea as human parasites in Palestine', *Parasitology*, 1 (1908), pp. 182-185.

Masterman, Ernest William Gurney, 'Hygiene and disease in Palestine in modern and in biblical times', *Palestine Exploration Quarterly*, 50 (1918), pp. 13-20, 56-71, 112-119; 51 (1919), pp. 27-36.

Masterman, Ernest William Gurney, 'Jerusalem from the point of view of health and disease', *Lancet*, (1918), pp. 305-307.

Masterman, Ernest William Gurney, 'Jerusalem from the sanitary point of view', *Home Words for Jerusalem* (1904).

Masterman, Ernest William Gurney, 'Jerusalem outside the walls', *Missionary Intelligence* (November 1895), pp. 174-175, 192-195.

Masterman, Ernest William Gurney, 'Miscellaneous notes made during a journey east and west of Jordan', *Palestine Exploration Quarterly*, 34 (1902), pp. 299-301.

Masterman, Ernest William Gurney, 'Notes and news', *Palestine Exploration Quarterly* 37 (1905).

Masterman, Ernest William Gurney, 'Notes from Damascus', *Palestine Exploration Quarterly*, 29 (1897), pp. 147-148.

Masterman, Ernest William Gurney, 'Notes of a visit to Engedy, Masada and Jebal Usdum', *Palestine Exploration Quarterly*, 40 (1908), pp. 229-244.

Masterman, Ernest William Gurney, 'Notes on some ruins and a rock-cut aqueduct in the wady Kumran', *Palestine Exploration Quarterly*, 35 (1903), pp. 264-267.

Masterman, Ernest William Gurney, 'Notes on some tropical diseases of Palestine', *Journal of Hygiene*, 13 (1913), pp. 49-62; 14 (1914), pp. 1-11.

Masterman, Ernest William Gurney, 'Observations on the Dead Sea Levels', *Palestine Exploration Quarterly*, 34 (1902), pp. 155-167, 297-301, 406-407; 35 (1903), pp. 177-178; 36 (1904), pp. 83-95, 163-168, 280-281; 37 (1905), pp. 158-161; 39 (1907), pp. 302-304; 40 (1908), pp. 160-161; 41 (1909), pp. 68-70.

Masterman, Ernest William Gurney, 'Palestine: its resources and suitability for colonization', *The Geographical Journal*, 50 (1917), pp. 12-26.

Masterman, Ernest William Gurney, 'Rodent ulcer', *St. Bartholomew's Hospital Report*, 29 (1893), pp. 189-201.

Masterman, Ernest William Gurney, 'Summary of observations on the rise and fall of the level of the Dead Sea. 1900-1913', *Palestine Exploration Quarterly*, 45 (1913), pp. 192-197.

Masterman, Ernest William Gurney, 'The cholera epidemic of last autumn in Palestine', *St. Bartholomew's Hospital Journal*, 10 (1903), pp. 62-63, 91-92.

Masterman, Ernest William Gurney, 'The Damascus railways', *Palestine Exploration Quarterly*, 29 (1897), pp. 198-200.

Masterman, Ernest William Gurney, 'The fisheries of Galilee', *Palestine Exploration Quarterly*, 40 (1908), pp. 40-51.

Masterman, Ernest William Gurney, 'The Galilee of Josephus, the Positions of Gabara, Jotapata and Taricheae', *Palestine Exploration Quarterly*, 42 (1910), pp. 268-280.

Masterman, Ernest William Gurney, 'The history of the Jerusalem Medicinal Mission', *Home Words for Jerusalem*, 41 (February 1911), published in: *Jewish Missionary Intelligence*, 1 (1911), pp. 12-14, 186.

Masterman, Ernest William Gurney, 'The new public health service in Palestine', *Palestine Exploration Quarterly*, 54 (1922), pp. 148-153.

Masterman, Ernest William Gurney, 'The recently-discovered aqueduct from the Virgins fountain', *Palestine Exploration Quarterly*, 34 (1902), pp. 35-38.

Masterman, Ernest William Gurney, 'The site of Capernaum', *Palestine Exploration Quarterly*, 39 (1907), pp. 220-229.

Masterman, Ernest William Gurney, 'The Trees and Shrubs of the Holy Land', *Palestine Exploration Quarterly*, 39 (1907), pp. 66-67.

Masterman, Ernest William Gurney, 'The water of Jacob's Well', *Palestine Exploration Quarterly*, 29 (1897), pp. 149-151.

Masterman, Ernest William Gurney, 'The water supply of Jerusalem, ancient and modern', *The Biblical World*, 19 (1902), pp. 87-112.

Masterman, Ernest William Gurney, 'Three cases of Addison's disease', *St. Bartholomew's Hospital Journal*, 29 (9) (1922), pp. 141-142.

Masterman, Ernest William Gurney, 'Two cases of spreading gangrene around the mouth occurring in adults', *St. Bartholomew's Hospital Report*, 27 (1891), pp. 205-210.

Masterman, Ernest William Gurney, 'Vine', in: J. Orr (ed.), *The International Standard Bible Encyclopedia* (Chicago, 1915).

Masterman, Ernest William Gurney, *Hygiene and Diseases in Palestine in Modern and Biblical Times* (London, 1919).

Masterman, Ernest William Gurney, *Studies in Galilee* (Chicago, 1909).

Masterman, Ernest William Gurney, *The Deliverance of Jerusalem* (London, New York, and Toronto, 1918).

Medical Register (London 1863, 1885).

Meyerhof, Max, 'A Short History of Ophthalmia during the Egyptian campaigns of 1798-1801', *The British Journal of Ophthalmology* (1932), p. 129-152.

Mirbach, Ernst Freiherr von (ed.), *Das deutsche Kaiserpaar im Heiligen Lande im Herbst 1898* (Berlin, 1899).

Morgenstern, Avraham, 'The First Jewish Hospital in Jerusalem', *Cathedra*, 33 (1984), pp. 107-124 [Hebrew].

Morgenstern, Avraham, *Lepers and Leprosy in Jerusalem: the Establishment of the German Leper Homes in the 19th Century* (M.A. thesis submitted to the University of Haifa 2006) [Hebrew].

Moussaieff, A., Frede, E., Amar, Z., Lev, E., Steinberg, D., Galily D. and Meshulam, R., 'The Jerusalem Balsam: From the Franciscan Monastery in the old city of Jerusalem to Martindale 33', *Journal of Ethnopharmacology*, 101 (2005), pp. 16-26.

Muehlens, Peter, 'Bericht über eine Malaria Expedition nach Jerusalem', *Zentralbl. f. Bakt*,. 69 (1913), pp. 41-85.

Muir, Ernest, 'Tiberias Hospital', *The Missionary Records of the United Free Church of Scotland*, 4 (1904).

Neuman, Bernard, *Die Heilige Stadt und deren Bewohner* (Hamburg, 1877).

Nicolayson, John, 'Mittheilungen für eine Skizze der Geschichte der englischen Mission und des evangelischen Bisthums zu Jerusalem', *Zions-Bote*, 1 (1852), pp. 6-16.

Nightingale, Florence, *The Institution of Kaiserswerth on the Rhine* (London, 1851).

Nissan, Shemuel and Martin, Petra, 'A proposal to Establish a Children Hospital in 19th Century Jerusalem: Dr. Max Sandreczky to the Grossherzog Friedrich Franz II', *Cathedra*, 107 (2003), pp. 167-182 [Hebrew].

Nissan, Shemuel and Martin, Petra, 'Max Sandreczky: A Pediatric Surgeon in 19th-Century Jerusalem', *Journal of Pediatric Surgery*, 33 (1998), pp. 1187-1193.

Olin, Stephan, *Travels in Egypt, Arabia Petraea, and the Holy Land*, 2 vols. (New York, 1843).

Oxford Dictionary of National Biography (Oxford, 2004).

Paxton, J.D., *Letters from Jerusalem* (London, 1839).

Perry, Yaron and Lev, Efraim, 'Dr Percy Charles Edward d'Erf Wheeler (1859-1944). A Notable Medical Missionary of the Holy Land', *Journal of Medical Biography* (in press).

Perry, Yaron and Lev, Efraim, 'Ernest William Gurney Masterman, British Physician and Scholar in the Holy Land', *Palestine Exploration Quarterly*, 138, 2(2006), pp. 133-146.

Perry, Yaron and Lev, Efraim, 'Nineteenth Century Medical Activities of the London Society for Promoting Christianity Amongst the Jews, in the Holy Land', *Medical History*, 47 (2003), pp. 67-88.

Perry, Yaron and Lev, Efraim, 'Walter Henry Anderson (1869-1937) the Holy Man of Safed', *Vesalius – Acta Internationalia Historiae Medicinae* (Forthcoming in 2007).

Perry, Yaron, 'Alexander, Michael Solomon (1799-1845), first bishop of the United Church of England and Ireland and of the Protestant Church of Germany in Jerusalem', *Oxford Dictionary of National Biography* (Oxford, 2004), vol 1, pp. 681-683.

Perry, Yaron, 'Anglo-German Cooperation in the Nineteenth-Century Jerusalem: The London Jew's Society and the Protestant Bishopric', *Jewish Culture and History*, 4 (2001), pp. 65-80.

Perry, Yaron, 'Blyth, George Francis Popham (1832-1914), bishop of Jerusalem and the East', *Oxford Dictionary of National Biography* (Oxford, 2004), vol 6, pp. 364-365.

Perry, Yaron, 'Gobat, Samuel (1799-1879), bishop in Jerusalem', *Oxford Dictionary of National Biography* (Oxford, 2004), vol. 22, p. 537.

Perry, Yaron, 'Tempelgesellschaft' (Deutscher Tempel)', *Religion in Geschichte und Gegenwart (RGG[4])* (Tübingen, 2005), vol. 8, pp. 154-155.

Perry, Yaron, 'The British Hospital in Safed', *Cathedra*, 103 (2002), pp. 69-84 [Hebrew].

Perry, Yaron, *British Mission to the Jews in Nineteenth-Century Palestine* (London, 2003).

Porush, E., *Sha'are Tsedek: To the History of the Hospital and its First Director* (Jerusalem, 1952) [Hebrew].

Preuss, Julius, *Biblical and Talmudic Medicine*, in: F. Rosner (trans.) (New York, 1983).

Qashani, Reuben, *Misgav Ladach, General Hospital in Jerusalem: 120 Years Anniversary* (Jerusalem, 1976).

Rabba, Yoel, *Erets Israel in the Descriptions of Russian pilgrims* (Jerusalem, 1987) [Hebrew].

Raz, Eli, *Dead Sea Book* (Jerusalem, 1993).

Reiche-Zeller, Lisl, *Johannes Zeller 1830-1902, Missionar in Palästina* (Stuttgart, 1987).

Rooker J., *Half-an-Hour in a… Jerusalem Dispensary*, A pamphlet published by the London Jews Society [1907], in: St. Albans.

Rubitschung, Otto, Das Deutsche Krankenhaus in Jaffa 1869 bis 1927 (Jerusalem, 1928).

Rubitschung, Otto, Der Werdegang des deutschen Krankenhauses in Jaffa (Jerusalem, 1927).

Ruppel, Hans-Rudolf (ed.), *Universeller Geist und guter Europäer. Christian Carl Josias von Bunsen 1791-1860* (Korbach, 1991).

Rushman, G.B., Davis, N.J. and Atkinson, R.S., *A Short History of Anaesthesia: The First 150 Years* (Oxford, 1996).

Sauer, Paul, *The Holy Land Called: The Story of the Temple Society* (Melbourne, 1991).

Sayce, A. Henry, 'The Ancient Hebrew Inscription in the Pool of Siloam', *Palestine Exploration Quarterly*, 13 (1881), pp. 282-285.

Schick, Conrad, 'Sonst und Jetzt. Die Veränderungen in Jerusalem und dem heiligen Lande in den letzten fünfzig Jahren', *Neueste Nachrichten aus dem Morgenlande*, 41 (1897), pp. 211-229.

Schischa, A., 'The Saga of 1855: A Study in Depth', in: S. and V.D. Lipman, *Century of Moses Montefiore* (Oxford, 1985), pp. 269-346.

Schittny, H.R., 'Die historische Apotheke der Franziskaner in Jerusalem', *Geschichte der Pharmazie*, 45 (1993), pp. 41–45.

Schmelz, Usiel Oskar, 'Some Demographic Peaculiarities of the Jews of Jerusalem in the Nineteenth Century', in: M. Maoz (ed.), *Studies on Palestine during the Ottoman Period* (Jerusalem, 1975). pp. 129-131.

Schmidt-Clausen, Kurt, *Vorweggenommene Einheit. Die Gründung des Bistums Jerusalem in Jahre 1841* (Berlin-Hamburg, 1965).

Schur, Nathan, 'Franciscan Physicians and Pharmacists in Jerusalem', in: Z. Amar, E. Lev and J. Schwartz (eds.), *Medicine in Jerusalem throughout the Ages* (Tel Aviv, 1999), pp. 99-105.

Schwacke, Norbert, 'The Austrian Hospital in Nazareth', in: M. Wrba (ed.), *Austrian Presence in the Holy Land in the 19th and Early 20th Century* (Tel Aviv, 1996), pp. 81-97.

Schwake, Norbert, 'Hospitals and European Colonial Policies in 19th and Early 20th Centuries', in: M. Wasserman and S. Kottek (eds.), *Health and Diseases in the Holy Land* (New York, 1996), pp. 231-262.

Schwake, Norbert, *Die Entwicklung des Krankenhauswesens der Stadt Jerusalem vom Ende des 18. bis zum Beginn des 20.Jahrhunderts* (Herzogenrath, 1983).

Scrimgeour, Frederic John, *Nazareth of To-day* (Edinburgh and London, 1913).

Seetzen, J. Ulrich, *Reisen durch Syrien, Palästina, etc.*, 2 vols. (Berlin, 1854).

Seidler, E., 'An historical survey of children's hospitals', in: L. Granshaw and R. Porter (eds.), *The Hospital in History* (London and New York, 1990). pp. 181-197.

Shell, E.H. and Masterman, Ernest William Gurney, 'A fatal case of anthrax infection by a shaving brush', *Lancet* (1916), p. 242.

Shilony, Zvi, 'The Activity of the Comte de Piéllat in Palestine (1884-1925)', *Cathedra*, 72 (1994), pp. 63-90 [Hebrew].

Shimkin, N., 'Trachoma in Palestine; its epidemiology and a review of measures for dealing with it', *British Journal of Ophthalmology* (1926), pp. 247-279.

Shvarts, Shifra, 'Messianism and politics in the establishment of Jewish Medical services in Jerusalem during the 19th century', In Z. Amar, E. Lev and J. Shwartz (eds.), *Medicine in Jerusalem throughout the ages* (Tell Aviv, 1999). pp. 129-146 [Hebrew].

Smith, George Adams, *Historical Geography of the Holy Land* (London, 1931).

Spyridon, S.N., 'Annals of Palestine 1821-1841', *Journal of the Palestine Oriental Society*, 18 (1938), pp. 63-152, in: *Extracts from Annals of Palestine 1821-1841, Manuscript – Monk Neophitos of Cyprus* (Jerusalem, 1979), pp. 18-28.

Stavrou, Theofanis George, *Russian Interests in Palestine 1882-1914. A study of Religious and Educational Enterprise* (Thessaloniki, 1963).

Stern Shimon, 'A Description of Medical Conditions in mid-19th-Century Jerusalem', in: Z. Amar, E. Lev and J. Schwartz (eds.), *Medicine in Jerusalem throughout the Ages* (Tel Aviv, 1999), pp. 107-127 [Hebrew].

Stern, Shimon, 'Titus Tobler, 19th Century Researcher of Eretz Israel', *Cathedra*, 48 (1998), pp. 30-45 [Hebrew].

Sticker, D. Anna, *Theodor Fliedner and Nursing* (Düsseldorf, 1972).

Still, Fredric George, *The History of Pediatrics* (London, 1965).

Stock, Eugene, *The History of the Church Missionary Society: Its Environment, Its Men and Its Work*, 3 vols. (London, 1899).

Stransky, Thomas, 'The Austrian Hospital at Tantur (1869-1918)', in: M. Wrba (ed.), *Austrian Presence in the Holy Land in the 19th and Early 20th Century* (Tel Aviv, 1996). pp. 98-121.

Strobel, August, *Conrad Schick. Ein Leben für Jerusalem* (Fürth, 1988).

Stuart, A. Moody, 'The Origin of the Mission', in: J.H. Wilson and J. Wells (eds.), *The Sea of Galilee Mission of the Free Church of Scotland* (Edinburgh and London, 1896).

Thiersch, W.J. Heinrich and Gobat, Samuel, *Samuel Gobat, Bishop of Jerusalem, His Life and Work* (London, 1884).

Tobler, Titus, *Beitrage zur Medizinischen Topographie von Jerusalem* (Berlin, 1855).

Tobler, Titus, *Denkblätter aus Jerusalem* (Konstanz, 1853).

Tobler, Titus, *Dritte Wanderung nach Palästina* (Gotha, 1859).

Tobler, Titus, *Nazareth in Palästina, nebst Anhang der vierten Wanderung* (Berlin, 1868).

Torrance, W. David. 'The Planting of the Mission in 1885', in: J.H. Wilson and J. Wells (eds.), *The Sea of Galilee Mission of the Free Church of Scotland* (Edinburgh and London, 1896).

Tsibkin, Vladimir, 'The Palestinian Imperial Pravoslavic Society (1882-1914)', *Cathedra*, 46 (1987), pp. 65-90 [Hebrew].

Ullmann, Manfred, *Islamic Medicine* (Edinburgh, 1978), pp. 1-6.

Ulman, Yesim Isil, 'The First Surgical Use of Chloroform in the Ottoman Empire', *The New History of Medicine Studies*, 5 (1999), pp. 87-94.

Underhill, H.W., 'Dead Sea levels and P.E.F. mark', *Palestine Exploration Quarterly*, 99 (1967), p. 45.

Veretė, Meir, 'The Restoration of the Jews in the Protestant Thought in England during the Years 1790-1840', *Zion*, 33 (1968), pp. 145-79 [Hebrew].

Volney, Constantin Francois, *Travels through Syria and Egypt in the Years 1783, 1784 &1785* (London, 1788).

Warren, Charles and Conder, Claude Reigneir, *The Survey of Western Palestine, Jerusalem* (London, 1884).

Warren, Charles, 'Copy of Letter Lost at es-Salt', *Palestine Exploration Quarterly*, (1869), pp. 13-14.

Watson, Gilbert, *Theriac and Mithridatium* (London, 1966).

Wells, J., 'The Deputation of 1884', in: J.H. Wilson and J. Wells (eds.), *The Sea of Galilee Mission of the Free Church of Scotland* (Edinburgh and London, 1896).

Wheeler, Percy d'Erf, 'Jerusalem Notes: Hospital Cleanings', *Jewish Missionary Intelligence* (1907), pp. 86-87.

Wheeler, Percy d'Erf, 'Malaria', *Palestine Exploration Quarterly*, 39 (1907), pp. 246-247; 40 (1908), pp. 86-87; 41 (1909), pp. 159-160.

Wheeler, Percy d'Erf, 'Visitation of the Sick in Jerusalem', *Jewish Missionary Intelligence* (1901), pp. 168-170.

Whitty, Irwine John, *Proposed Water Supply and Sewerage for Jerusalem* (London, 1863).

Wilkinson J., *The Coogate Doctors, The History of the Edinburgh Medical Missionary Society 1841-1991* (Edinburgh, 1991).

Wilson, Charles William and Warren, Charles, *The Recovery of Jerusalem* (Jerusalem, 1871).

Wilson, Charles William, *Ordnance Survey of Jerusalem made in the year 1864 to 1865* (Southampton, 1866).

Wilson, G., 'The History of the Hospital', in: J.H. Wilson and J. Wells (eds.), *The Sea of Galilee Mission of the Free Church of Scotland* (Edinburgh and London, 1896).

Wilson, H., 'The Revival of the Original Proposal in 1883', in: J.H. Wilson and J. Wells (eds.), *The Sea of Galilee Mission of the Free Church of Scotland* (Edinburgh and London, 1896).

Wolff, Philipp, 'Rückblicke auf die jüngste Geschichte Jerusalems von Jahre 1856 bis 1866', *Sieben Artikel über Jerusalem aus den Jahren 1859 bis 1869* (Stuttgart, 1869).

Woodville, Wilson, *Medical Botany* 3 vols. (London, 1819).

Ya'ari, Abraham, *Igrot Eretz Israel* [Letters of the Land of Israel] (Tel Aviv, 1943) [Hebrew].

Yekutiel, Perez, 'Masterman, Muehlens and Malaria, Jerusalem 1912-1913', *Korot*, 12 (1996-1997), pp. 107-123.

Ziadat, Adel, 'Western Medicine in Palestine, 1860-1940: The Edinburgh Medical Missionary Society and its Hospital', *Canadian Bulletin of Medical History*, 10 (1993), pp. 269-279.

INDEX